I strongly recommend Dr. Ozner's book, *The Miami Mediterranean Diet*, for anyone who is interested in living a long and healthy life. This book is a concise, no-nonsense approach for heart disease prevention. With so many fad diets that are here today and gone tomorrow, finally there is a clinically proven and sensible approach, as Dr. Ozner provides practical dietary and lifestyle guidelines for defeating heart disease.

—BARRY T. KATZEN, MD
Medical Director, Baptist Cardiac & Vascular Institute of Miami

---

The current medical literature is replete with articles confirming what Dr. Ozner has been advocating for many years—that prevention is the best treatment for heart disease. In his book, *The Miami Mediterranean Diet*, he outlines a strategy that, combined with an exercise program, has allowed me to reduce my weight, my blood pressure, and my cholesterol. I have a greater sense of well-being and I feel that I will live a longer and healthier life.

—JERROLD YOUNG, MD

In *The Miami Mediterranean Diet*, Dr. Michael Ozner not only makes a compelling argument for the importance of the Mediterranean diet and lifestyle for overall health, but gives a comprehensive guide for ways to incorporate this diet into all of our lives. Research has clearly shown that those who follow a life-long Mediterranean diet and lifestyle are giving themselves the best insurance for a healthy life and now Dr. Ozner brings that to our shores.

—RANDOLPH P. MARTIN, MD
Director of Noninvasive Cardiology, Emory University Hospital

---

A valuable resource from preventive cardiologist Michael Ozner providing heart healthy dietary information, sample meal plans, and an exciting array of recipes.

—NANETTE K. WENGER, MD
Professor of Medicine (Cardiology),
Emory University School of Medicine

This book is a direct path to the visceral pleasure of well-prepared food and cardiovascular health. *The Miami Mediterranean Diet* provides a sane alternative to the faddist and extremist diets that lead to short-term weight loss and long-term weight gain."

—JOSEPH L. IZZO, JR., MD
Professor of Medicine & Pharmacology, State University of New York at Buffalo Clinical Director of Medicine, Erie County Medical Center, Buffalo, New York

———

I wholeheartedly endorse the Mediterranean diet, a way of eating that has been in existence for thousands of years. *The Miami Mediterranean Diet* is based on this way of life, encouraging a balanced, well-nourished food plan including whole grains, fresh fruits and vegetables, and lower fat intake. Following Ozner's stated food plan, coupled with caloric control and daily exercise, can lead to both weight loss and a healthy heart. The recipes are easy to produce and generate delicious meals; no one would feel deprived adhering to the stated plan.

—KAREN LIEBERMAN, PhD, RD
Professor and Chair, the Hospitality College,
Johnson & Wales University, Florida Campus

———

I have bounced from one diet to another, including the "low carb" diets. My weight would go up and down on these fad diets and I felt that I was mortgaging my long-term health in order to achieve weight loss. I adopted Dr. Ozner's dietary and lifestyle guidelines and I have achieved my goal— controlled and steady weight loss. In addition, my cholesterol has dropped, my blood pressure has normalized, and I have more energy. I highly endorse this book for anyone seeking to decrease their risk of heart disease and improve their overall health.

—PATIENT (CP)

EXPANDED   EDITION

LOSE WEIGHT AND
LOWER YOUR RISK OF HEART DISEASE
WITH 300 DELICIOUS RECIPES

The Miami
Mediterranean
Diet

*Lifesaving Advice Based on the Clinically
Proven Mediterranean Diet and Lifestyle*

Michael Ozner, MD
MEDICAL DIRECTOR
Cardiovascular Prevention Institute of South Florida

BENBELLA BOOKS, INC.
Dallas, Texas

BenBella Books, Inc.
10300 N. Central Expressway, Suite 400
Dallas, TX 75231
Send feedback to feedback@benbellabooks.com
www.benbellabooks.com

Printed in the United States of America
10 9 8 7 6 5 4

Library of Congress Cataloging-in-Publication Data is available for this title.
ISBN 978-1933771-65-6

Proofreading by Stacia Seaman, Emily Chauvier, Maggie McGuire, & Erica Lovett
Front cover by Todd Michael Bushman • Full cover design by Laura Watkins
Design and composition by John Reinhardt Book Design
Index by Shoshana Hurwitz
Printed by Bang Printing

Distributed by Perseus Distribution
(www.perseusdistribution.com)

To place orders through Perseus Distribution:
Tel: 800-343-4499
Fax: 800-351-5073
E-mail: orderentry@perseusbooks.com

Significant discounts for bulk sales are available.
Please contact Glenn Yeffeth at glenn@benbellabooks.com or (214) 750-3628.

Acknowledgments

I would like to thank my patients and colleagues who have given me the inspiration and motivation to write *The Miami Mediterranean Diet*.

I am especially grateful to the following individuals who have taken extensive time and effort to review and critique *The Miami Mediterranean Diet*: Barry T. Katzen, MD, a pioneer in interventional radiology and Medical Director of the Baptist Cardiac & Vascular Institute at Baptist Hospital of Miami; Randolph P. Martin, MD, Director of Noninvasive Cardiology at Emory University in Atlanta; and Karen Lieberman, PhD, RD, Professor and Chair of the Hospitality College at Johnson & Wales University, Florida Campus. I would also like to thank Nanette K. Wenger, MD, and Joseph L. Izzo, MD, for reviewing and commenting on *The Miami Mediterranean Diet*.

I would like to express my gratitude to all of the nurse educators who share my passion for cardiovascular disease prevention, and who have helped me organize and promote the Wellness & Prevention Program at the Baptist Cardiac & Vascular Institute at Baptist Hospital of Miami. This program provides education and prevention strategies for patients who have heart disease or diabetes and for those with risk factors for cardiovascular disease.

I am also grateful to Glenn Yeffeth, Leah Wilson, and Laura Watkins at BenBella Books for their steadfast guidance and advice.

Finally, and most importantly, I would like to thank my wife, Christine Ozner, RN, who has a special interest in nutrition and Mediterranean cooking and has contributed immensely to the writing and editing of this book.

To my wife, Christine, and my children, Jennifer and Jonathan:
You are my heart and soul.

Congratulations! By reading this book and following the principles of the Miami Mediterranean diet and lifestyle, you will begin to take charge of your cardiovascular health.

This book is intended to provide information on cardiovascular disease prevention. However, it is *not* intended to replace the doctor-patient relationship. I recommend that you discuss all prevention and treatment options with your personal treating physician. Regular office visits between a patient and his or her doctor to discuss cardiovascular prevention strategies provide the optimum approach in the ongoing battle against heart disease.

Contents

Appendices

Foreword

We are at war in the United States of America, and our enemy is quite formidable. It has killed more people than all of the wars which we have previously fought. Every thirty seconds it claims another victim. We have identified this enemy but we have not defeated it.

Its name is cardiovascular disease.

Is there a solution? Can we defeat cardiovascular disease and its manifestations (heart attack, stroke, peripheral vascular disease)?

The answer is yes! First, we must realize that our most effective weapon is prevention, not intervention. Prevention strategies must begin at an early age and continue for life. Proper diet, exercise, stress management, the cessation of smoking, and appropriate medical therapies are the weapons most needed in our ongoing battle against heart disease.

It is my hope that this book will provide you with the information that you need to begin an effective prevention strategy. Don't sit back and wait for this silent killer to strike. Take action before you develop symptoms. Defeat cardiovascular disease and live a long, happy, and heart-healthy life.

PART ONE

THE MIAMI MEDITERRANEAN DIET AND LIFESTYLE

How Your Diet and Lifestyle Are Affecting Your Health

Ted and Giovanni

It was a typical day for Ted. He awoke at 6 A.M. and had his usual breakfast of bacon, eggs, and fried potatoes. He left home in a hurry after an argument with his wife and drove to his office to begin another stressful day as a real estate executive. At a 9:30 A.M. board meeting, he presented a proposal for purchasing a large office complex. During the meeting he had coffee and doughnuts, and smoked several cigarettes. It was customary for Ted to argue with his partners, and today was no different. After several phone calls he was off to the airport to catch a noon flight. He had no time to sit down for lunch, so he went to his favorite fast food drive-through for a burger and fries, which he ate quickly on the way to the airport. After parking his car and walking briskly to the terminal, he felt a crushing chest pain and broke into a sweat. He grabbed a roll of Tums from his pocket and chewed several tablets. The pain subsided briefly, only to return with a vengeance several minutes later. This time the pain was an intense sensation of pressure in his chest that radiated out to his arms and his jaw. He collapsed at the security gate and lost consciousness. When he awoke, he was in a nearby emergency room, having been resuscitated by paramedics. It was clear that Ted had suffered a massive heart attack and was lucky to be alive. Following an extensive hospital stay including heart catheterization and coronary bypass surgery, Ted's life would never be the same.

Giovanni awoke the same day in his small Italian village. He ate a light breakfast of whole grain bread with jam and fruit. He walked to his nearby office and passed a pleasant morning with his clients in his import/export business. At 2:00 P.M., he returned home, where he shared an enjoyable lunch with his family and friends. Lunch consisted of a salad with olive oil, whole wheat pasta, whole grain bread with garlic, goat cheese, red wine, and fresh fruit. Following lunch, he rested for an hour, and then returned to work.

Was Ted's heart attack preventable? Is Giovanni's good health a matter of luck? Or are both the consequences of diet and lifestyle?

The Toxic American Diet and Lifestyle

The American diet and lifestyle are toxic. Our food is contaminated with pesticides and preservatives, and contains an excessive amount of dangerous fats, sugars, and salt. We no longer exercise and our lives are plagued by chronic stress. In the last fifty years, there's been an explosive rise in heart disease, stroke, high blood pressure, diabetes, and obesity, diseases that have been directly linked to the food we eat and the lifestyle we lead.

We have been led to believe that the solution to this epidemic is to be found in medical or surgical intervention: in prescription medications and invasive surgeries. But despite the billions of dollars we spend on health care, we continue to suffer and die unnecessarily from diseases *that can be prevented*.

I have been practicing preventive cardiology for more than twenty-five years, and have helped countless numbers of patients discover the real secret of long-term health: the optimal nutrition and healthy daily practices of the Miami Mediterranean diet and lifestyle.

Heart Disease: Your First Symptom May Be Your Last

Why do I practice preventive cardiology? Because heart disease is the number one killer of men and women in America and in most developed countries around the world—and most people never see it coming.

It would be nice if we had a warning system that alerted us to heart disease. Many people think chest pain is that warning system. Unfortunately, for the majority of men and women, the first symptom you experience is a heart attack—or sudden death. By then, it's too late.

In many respects, coronary heart disease is a silent killer—we are completely unaware of its presence in our body until a plaque ruptures and a heart attack occurs. Recent data has revealed that small plaques (which cause no symptoms) are in fact *more* likely than large plaques to suddenly rupture and lead to a heart attack or sudden death. The only way to defeat this formidable enemy, cardiovascular disease, is to attack when the enemy is most easily defeated—prior to the onset of symptoms!

The Mediterranean diet has been shown to reduce the risk of:

- Allergies
- Alzheimer's disease
- Arthritis
- Asthma
- Cancer
- Chronic obstructive lung disease
- Depression
- Diabetes
- High blood pressure
- High cholesterol
- Inflammatory bowel disease
- Metabolic syndrome

Believing in preventive cardiology doesn't mean I think surgery is never a necessary step. There are absolutely situations where surgical or cardiac catheterization procedures are not only needed but may save lives, especially in the case of patients with "unstable" heart disease, meaning they have an impending heart attack or are actually experiencing one. However, the vast majority of patients a doctor sees in his or her office are not unstable. Rather, they are stable patients who either have risk factors for coronary heart disease or have "stable" blockages in their arteries. And too often, doctors rely on coronary artery bypass surgery and coronary stent placement when the best treatment for the patient is aggressive prevention, which can halt the progression of cardiovascular disease and potentially even reverse it.

Through my practice, I've learned that prevention is more important than medication or bypass surgery in achieving greater heart health. And together, diet and lifestyle can reduce or eliminate the need for expensive medications and risky surgical interventions.

Susan's Story

About four and a half years ago, I awoke at about 5 A.M. with the most horrible pain in my chest and extreme shortness of breath. In a panic, and with an unbelievable sense of impending doom, I woke my husband, who immediately called 911. Forty thousand dollars later, through the grace of God, I had survived a major heart attack.

Seven months earlier, I had experienced a few minor symptoms that led me to see a group of doctors. They did some tests, performed a heart procedure to put a stent in one of my coronary arteries, and told me that I could go home and relax, because they had "taken care" of my problem. After my heart attack, those same doctors told me that I was "stable" now that they had put in a second stent, but that I should return to the emergency room if I experienced any more chest pain. I realized that I needed to do more than just wait for the next heart attack to occur. I needed to take steps personally that would help me avoid another such experience, or worse. I have two grown children and three adorable grandkids. I desperately want to be around to enjoy them and to spend those coveted golden years with my husband. There had to be more that could be done. I felt it was just a matter of time before I once again found myself lying on an ER stretcher, praying that I would survive. The word "despondent" barely describes my anxiety.

I was determined to learn more about heart disease and what my options were. A few months later, my husband learned about a cardiologist in Miami who exclusively practiced cardiovascular prevention. We learned that Dr. Ozner gave lectures on heart disease prevention to other physicians as well as to the general public. After doing some research, I began to feel there was hope for me, so I made an appointment to see him.

Dr. Ozner started me on the Miami Mediterranean diet and a regime of medical therapy to lower my cholesterol and blood pressure. He also started me on a walking program. When Dr. Ozner first mentioned lifestyle changes and diet, I became concerned; I had tried other diets, but after the initial weight loss I would eventually gain the weight back. I began to realize that those diets didn't make much sense. Dr. Ozner told me he had based the Miami Mediterranean diet on a way of eating that has been in existence for thousands of years, and has been proven over the last fifty years to reduce heart disease risk.

I've lost a lot of weight on the Miami Mediterranean diet and now maintain a normal weight. This is a diet I can live with for the rest of my life! As a matter of fact, it's a way of life that my entire family can embrace; my entire family now follows the diet and exercise program.

As for me, I haven't needed any more cardiac procedures and I feel better than I have in years!

Beyond Heart Disease Prevention

But this isn't just about heart disease. The Miami Mediterranean diet and lifestyle lowers the risk of a multitude of chronic diseases. You may very well wonder how a single eating plan can afford all these benefits. That's a fair question. The secret seems to lie in the fact that the Mediterranean diet is *synergistic*. This means that the components are not only nutritious in themselves, but when combined with one another, act together to provide added benefits. They are more powerful in combination than if they were eaten separately.

The Miami Mediterranean diet is full of fruits and vegetables rich in antioxidants, which help prevent the damage to your body's cells that cause heart disease, cancer, and other diseases. The diet also features whole grain foods rich in fiber, which has been shown to help balance cholesterol and also prevent some forms of cancer. In addition, the diet decreases inflammation, which has been strongly linked to the development of heart disease, cancer, and other ailments such as arthritis.

In short, if you're looking for a diet that will benefit your entire body, you can do no better than to choose the Miami Mediterranean diet.

The Miami Mediterranean Diet and Lifestyle

The Miami Mediterranean Diet

The Mediterranean diet—a diet of whole non-processed foods, rich in a wide variety of health-promoting vitamins and nutrients—is the ideal dietary plan for long-term heart health and weight control; multiple clinical trials have demonstrated its beneficial impact.

A brief summary of some of the important ones:

The Seven Countries Study

This landmark twenty-year study by Dr. Ancel Keys demonstrated that a diet low in saturated animal fat and processed food was associated with a low incidence of mortality from coronary heart disease and cancer. Beginning in the late 1950s, the study followed almost 13,000 men from seven different countries (Italy, Greece, Yugoslavia, Netherlands, Finland, United States, and Japan). Men living in the Mediterranean region had the lowest incidence of heart disease and the longest life expectancy. And Greek men had a 90% lower likelihood of premature death from heart attack compared to American men!

The Lyon Diet Heart Study

This study compared a Mediterranean diet to a control diet resembling the American Heart Association Step 1 diet in heart attack survivors, and found that, compared to the American Heart Association Step 1 diet, the Mediterranean diet afforded significantly better protection against recurrent heart attacks and death. The Mediterranean diet was associated with a 70% decreased risk of death and a 73% decreased risk of recurrent cardiac events.

The DART Study
This study of over 2,000 men who had suffered heart attacks tested the hypothesis that fatty fish such as salmon and tuna, rich in omega-3 fatty acids, are protective against coronary heart disease. The results demonstrated that a modest intake of fatty fish twice per week (around 300 grams per week) reduced the risk of coronary heart disease death by 32% and overall death by 29%.

The Singh Indo-Mediterranean Diet Study
This study placed 499 patients with risk factors for coronary heart disease on an Indo-Mediterranean diet rich in fruits, vegetables, whole grains, walnuts, and almonds. The study found that the diet change resulted in a reduction in serum cholesterol and was associated with a significant reduction in heart attack and sudden cardiac death. Subjects were also found to have fewer cardiovascular events than those on a conventional diet.

The Alzheimer's Disease Study
This study by Dr. Nikolaos Scarmeas and colleagues from Columbia University Medical Center in New York demonstrated that a Mediterranean diet reduced the risk of developing Alzheimer's disease by 68%. Another study from this same group showed that patients with Alzheimer's disease who followed a Mediterranean diet had reduced mortality.

The Metabolic Syndrome Study
This study by Dr. Katherine Esposito and colleagues from Italy evaluated the effects of a Mediterranean diet on patients with metabolic syndrome (obesity, elevated blood sugar, elevated blood pressure, abnormal cholesterol profile, and markers of vascular inflammation). A Mediterranean diet was shown to improve all of the components of the metabolic syndrome.

Why does the Mediterranean diet lower the risk of death from heart disease and cancer compared to an American or Western diet? There are many theories. Scientific studies have linked the intake of saturated fat and trans fat to the development of heart disease and other diseases, including cancer. The consumption of saturated fat is limited in the Mediterranean diet, and trans fats are not present. This is in stark contrast with the typical Western or American diet, which contains an excessive amount of saturated fat and trans fat. Many of the foods present in the Mediterranean diet have been shown to decrease inflammation, and current research has demonstrated the pivotal role that inflammation plays in the development and progression of heart disease, cancer, diabetes, and an increasing list of other diseases. In contrast, the typical American (Western) diet, with its high levels of saturated fat, trans fat, and omega-6 fat, promotes inflammation and increases the incidence of heart disease and a multitude of other diseases initiated and aggravated by a state of chronic inflammation.

Whatever the reasons, I have witnessed the diet's success over and over again in my Miami cardiovascular disease prevention practice. And by adapting the traditional Mediterranean diet to our modern lifestyle, I have created a delicious and easy diet for long-term health that I call the Miami Mediterranean diet.

How has the traditional Mediterranean diet been adapted? Nutritional science has introduced new and exciting ways to cook and prepare food. For instance, newly developed non-hydrogenated buttery spreads are a great, healthier replacement for butter or margarine in cooking and baking (they contain no trans fats and support heart health by providing omega-3 fat and plant sterols). Another example is the introduction of pomegranate juice, which has recently been shown to lower blood pressure and help reverse the build-up of fatty deposits (atherosclerosis) in our arteries. Nevertheless, the basics of a traditional Mediterranean diet remain unchanged: a wide variety of fresh whole non-processed foods, frequently enjoyed with a glass of wine in a relaxed setting with family and friends.

Let's take a look at the main components of the Mediterranean diet and their chief health benefits.

Whole grains

Whole (non-refined) grains are an integral part of the Mediterranean diet, and have been shown to decrease the risk of heart disease, diabetes, and cancer. A whole grain kernel consists of an outer layer, the bran (fiber); a middle layer (complex carbohydrates and protein); and an inner layer (vitamins, minerals, and protein). The process of refining, common outside the Mediterranean region, destroys the outer and inner layer of the grain, resulting in grains that lack fiber and disease-fighting vitamins and phytochemicals. Examples of whole grains that are common to the Mediterranean diet are oatmeal, kasha, quinoa, and barley.

Fresh Fruits and Vegetables

Go to any market in the Mediterranean basin and you will find a bountiful supply of fresh, native fruits and vegetables. Fruits and vegetables contain an abundance of vitamins, minerals, fiber, and complex carbohydrates that lower the risk of heart disease and cancer. In particular, phytonutrients, concentrated in the skin of fruits and vegetables, are powerful plant-derived nutrients that help fight disease and improve our health. It is recommended that we eat a wide variety of colors (oranges, blueberries, red apples, spinach, yellow squash, etc.) in order to get all the nutritional benefits that fruits and vegetables can provide.

Nuts

Nuts, like olive oil, have been an essential part of the Mediterranean diet since antiquity. Nuts such as almonds and walnuts are rich in monounsaturated fat and omega-3 fatty acids, as well as being good sources of protein, fiber, and vitamins. Nuts are an excellent snack that can assist with weight loss thanks to their high satiety. Several clinical trials have demonstrated that regular nut consumption leads to lower cholesterol, lower risk of coronary heart disease, and a significant reduction in the risk of heart attack.

Beans (Legumes)

Beans are also consumed on a regular basis in the Mediterranean region, and are a rich source of soluble and insoluble fiber, which help curb appetite and reduce cholesterol. In addition, beans are an excellent source of protein and vitamins. Regular bean consumption lowers the risk of heart disease, cancer, and diabetes.

Fish

Oily fish, prevalent in the Mediterranean diet, provide us with a rich source of protein and omega-3 fatty acids. Omega-3 fatty acids have a favorable impact on cholesterol and triglyceride levels, and reduce the risk of heart attack. They also help to reduce inflammation and, with regular consumption, decrease the risk of sudden death due to fatal cardiac arrhythmias.

A warning: Several species of fish may contain high levels of mercury and other contaminants, so pregnant women and young children should exercise caution. Nevertheless, for most adults, the cardiovascular benefits of fish consumption outweigh the risks, especially if you choose fish varieties that provide the highest amount of omega-3 fatty acids and tend to contain the lowest amount of mercury. The best choices are salmon, albacore tuna, herring, sardines, shad, trout, flounder, and pollock. Avoid tilefish, swordfish, shark, and king mackerel, as these fish species tend to have the highest mercury content.

Olive Oil

Olive oil, made by crushing and then pressing olives, is the "soul" of the Mediterranean diet, and provides the taste and flavor that is so much a part of Mediterranean dishes. It is rich in monounsaturated fat—the type of fat which is beneficial for heart health.

The regular use of olive oil instead of butter or margarine is associated with a reduced risk of heart disease, cancer, diabetes, and inflammatory disorders like asthma and arthritis. Olive oil also has a favorable impact on cholesterol. Besides decreasing total cholesterol, it also lowers bad (LDL) cholesterol, and makes our bodies less susceptible to oxidative damage by free radicals. Olive oil also helps maintain or increase good (HDL) cholesterol, so the total cholesterol to HDL cholesterol ratio (an important key to cholesterol health) is improved.

In addition, olive oil can help you lose weight. A study in Boston showed that a diet which included olive oil and nuts resulted in sustained weight loss over eighteen months compared to a low-fat diet. People also stayed on the diet longer because they did not feel deprived.

Red Wine

Moderate alcohol consumption has been shown to lower the risk of coronary heart disease, and red wine, often part of a Mediterranean meal, is believed to have several advantages over other forms of alcohol. Red wine contains polyphenols and resveratrol, two substances that help to promote heart health. Resveratrol, a powerful antioxidant, is more abundant in red wine than white wine; it lowers the bad (LDL) cholesterol and raises the good (HDL) cholesterol, and also has a beneficial impact on clotting.

Remember, alcohol should be consumed in moderation: wine consumption should not exceed one to two (5-ounce) glasses per day. For those individuals who do not wish to consume wine, grape juice is an excellent alternative: grape juice—specifically purple grape juice—also lowers the risk of heart attack. Since most heart attacks occur in the morning, many patients with cardiovascular risk factors often have a small glass of purple grape juice with breakfast.

The Miami Mediterranean Diet Pyramid

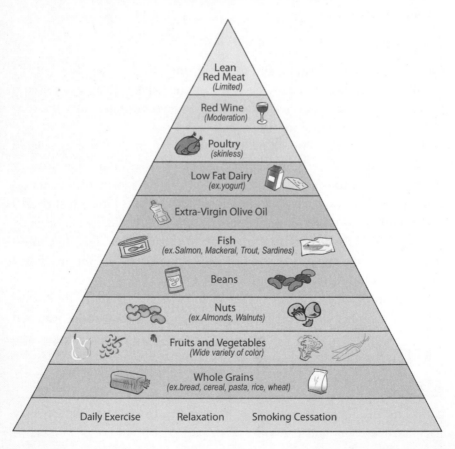

Lean Red Meat (Limited)

Red Wine (Moderation)

Poultry (skinless)

Low Fat Dairy (ex.yogurt)

Extra-Virgin Olive Oil

Fish (ex.Salmon, Mackeral, Trout, Sardines)

Beans

Nuts (ex.Almonds, Walnuts)

Fruits and Vegetables (Wide variety of color)

Whole Grains (ex.bread, cereal, pasta, rice, wheat)

Daily Exercise   Relaxation   Smoking Cessation

The Miami Mediterranean Lifestyle

You'll notice that, in the anecdote I used to open the book, Giovanni's day differed from Ted's in more than just diet. The pace of Giovanni's day was more relaxed—yet more active!—with more room for enjoyment. It is important not just what you eat, but the circumstances in which you eat it, and the way you live between meals!

Stress: The Silent Killer

People living in Mediterranean countries tend to have less stress in their daily lives compared to their American counterparts. They spend more time enjoying their meals with family and friends. They often relax and take a short nap after lunch. A recent study showed that a regular midday nap reduced the risk of death from heart disease by 37%!

Often, doctors don't discuss the deleterious impact of chronic stress on long-term health with patients during routine office visits. This does not mean that stress is not an important risk factor—indeed, it may be the most important! The problem with stress is that it cannot be measured the way cholesterol or blood pressure can. In addition, what causes stress for one person may not cause stress for another. I am reminded of a story I once heard about two matadors from Spain. Pepe and Poncho were having lunch before a bullfight. Pepe said, "Poncho, isn't this great? I love bullfighting. I live to enter the stadium and fight the bull in front of all those people." Poncho replied, "That's great, Pepe, but I hate what I do for a living—I have constant nightmares of been gored by the bull, and my stomach is tied up in knots for days before each fight." Here are two men in the same profession with completely opposite views regarding the stress it causes.

Chronic stress increases stress hormones, such as cortisol and adrenaline, which in turn increase blood pressure, cause the heartbeat to become rapid, and increase the likelihood of forming blood clots. Studies have shown that chronic stress significantly increases the risk of heart attack. To make matters worse, those individuals who are "hot reactors"—who have a short fuse, are impatient, and have a high hostility index—are especially prone to cardiovascular calamities.

What, then, is the treatment for stress? First, let's be realistic—we all have periods of stress in our lives. Some of us, unfortunately, have more stress than others. Regardless, the first step in handling stress is to take a realistic view of the factors responsible for stress in our lives and try our best to modify them. Next, I recommend a physical exercise program—not because exercise eliminates stress, but rather because people who exercise are better able to handle stress. There is a physiological explanation for the beneficial effects of exercise on stress: people who engage in regular aerobic exercise have lower catecholamine levels—in other words, their adrenaline levels are lower and rise less dramatically with stressful situations. In addition to a regular exercise program, I encourage my patients to begin relaxation response training, yoga, self-hypnosis, or meditation. Finally, prayer offers significant stress reduction for some individuals. If these lifestyle changes do not result in a significant reduction in stress, then a consultation with a psychologist or psychiatrist may be appropriate.

---

10 Steps for Stress Reduction

- Exercise daily
- Meditate
- Pray
- Enjoy a close relationship with family and friends
- Set realistic goals in life
- Live within your means
- Try yoga
- Enjoy hobbies and interests outside of your work
- Have a postitive outlook on life and never lose your sense of humor
- Laugh, smile, and enjoy your life!

Exercise Daily—Your Heart Will Thank You

Daily exercise is an integral part of the Miami Mediterranean lifestyle, and it does more than just help you handle stress. Whether it's walking to the market or working in the garden, regular daily exercise is essential for good health. Exercise raises good (HDL) cholesterol, lowers blood pressure, and optimizes bone health, reducing the risk of osteoporosis. Regular exercise also provides a sense of well-being. Physical inactivity, along with poor dietary habits, has led to an epidemic of obesity in America. And several studies have shown that being unfit is even more deleterious to our health than being overweight. Unfortunately, we have become a nation of "couch potatoes." Getting people to exercise is difficult. We use the elevator instead of stairs; we ride in golf carts instead of walking; we park as close as possible to the store in order to walk the fewest number of steps.

The solution is to incorporate exercise into our daily activities. Exercise does not necessarily mean jogging five miles a day; simply walking for thirty minutes a day has been shown to decrease the risk of heart attack and cardiovascular death. The benefits of regular aerobic exercise are significant. Besides the benefits listed above, a regular exercise program will also reduce fatigue and improve lung function. And adding resistance training with light weights can improve bone health further and help maintain muscle tone.

---

5 Easy Exercise Tips

- Walk in place for thirty minutes while watching your favorite TV show—get off the couch!
- Park farther away from your destination (office, store, etc.) and enjoy a short walk
- Climb stairs instead of using the elevator
- Walk for the initial part of your lunch break, before eating lunch
- Use a pedometer—strive for 10,000 steps per day

The Ten Commandments of the Miami Mediterranean Diet and Lifestyle

1. Eat a wide variety of fresh, non-processed food
2. Avoid saturated fat, trans fat, refined sugar, and excess sodium
3. Substitute olive oil or trans fat–free vegetable spreads for margarine or butter
4. Limit portion size
5. Drink an adequate amount of water
6. If you consume alcohol, do so in moderation
7. Exercise daily (minimum thirty minutes per day)

8. Abstain from smoking
9. Relax (especially after meals)
10. Never lose your sense of humor—laugh, smile, and enjoy life!

Why Choose the Miami Mediterranean Diet?

What Is Wrong with the Popular Fad Diets?

Americans have always been enamored with "quick fix" diets that promise rapid, sustained weight loss. The problem with these diets is that they have no scientific basis, and there is no long-term data demonstrating their effectiveness regarding sustained weight loss or long-term health.

I consider these diets to be fad diets. Fad diets usually promise quick and easy weight loss, but the sad truth is that, although some of these diets may result in initial weight loss, the weight is quickly gained back. That initial weight loss is often not healthy weight loss, either. Starving yourself can also lead to weight loss, but it deprives you of the vitamins and nutrients you need to live, and can do permanent damage to your body.

Here's a round-up of some popular diets and their drawbacks:

- *Low-fat diets (Ornish and Pritikin)*: These low-fat, high-carbohydrate, and mainly vegetarian diets are hard to follow, and not palatable for most Americans.
- *AHA (American Heart Association) diet*: This low-fat diet can lead to decreased good (HDL) cholesterol, and heart disease may progress regardless. The AHA diet contains less monounsaturated fat and omega-3 fat than the Mediterranean diet, and is associated with a higher risk of heart attack and death; the Lyon Heart Study demonstrated a 73%

reduction in cardiovascular endpoints (heart attack or death) in patients following a Mediterranean diet rather than an AHA Step 1 diet.

- *Low-carbohydrate diets (Atkins and South Beach)*: There is no long-term data demonstrating clinical benefit of following these diets, and concern about increasing the risk of heart disease and cancer make low-carbohydrate diets suspect according to many doctors. These diets are high in protein and saturated fat, and restrict carbohydrates. They do often lead to a quick, early drop in weight due to water loss, but this process of water loss can result in fluid and electrolyte changes that may lead to serious cardiac arrhythmias (heart rhythm disturbances) and kidney malfunction. The impact of these diets on cholesterol levels is unpredictable. Eating an excessive amount of saturated fat while following these diets causes some people to experience a significant rise in their bad (LDL) cholesterol—especially if they absorb cholesterol at a higher-than-average rate.

  Low-carbohydrate diets that achieve an "artificial" weight loss due to water loss from glycogen breakdown and ketosis (a condition that occurs when there is a lack of carbohydrates in the diet) are usually not effective in the long run. They are, however, potentially more dangerous, which is why many doctors do not recommend them. Some of the reported side effects and complications of these diets include a potential increased risk of:

  - Cancer
  - Cardiac arrhythmia (disorder of the heart rhythm)
  - Coronary heart disease
  - Deficiency of micronutrients
  - Dehydration
  - Diabetes
  - Elevated cholesterol
  - Elevated CRP (a marker of inflammation)
  - Gout
  - Halitosis (bad breath)
  - Impaired cognitive (memory) function
  - Kidney malfunction
  - Kidney stones
  - Optic neuropathy

Juan's Story

I have always been a quick-fix weight loss junkie, and jumped from one fad diet to another. It's not that I didn't take these diets seriously; I did. I tried protein shakes, miracle pills, and low-carb diets. The Atkins and South Beach diets really sounded good to me because you could eat as much as you wanted, and still have a few carbs and a variety of meat without having to worry about portion size or exercise. What could be better? At first I lost sixteen pounds. Fabulous! The only trouble was that I regained the weight. It became a vicious cycle. Sadly, I finally realized that these diets just didn't work.

I knew I had to do something that would actually work. I'm only thirty-eight, and even though I was overweight, I was otherwise healthy. But I have a strong family history of heart disease. My father had a heart attack early in life, and he died at the age of fifty-two from a second one. My uncle had a stroke, and subsequently died of a heart attack when he was sixty-one. My aunt has diabetes, and my sister, who is overweight, was recently diagnosed with it as well.

Because of my family history, I went to see Dr. Ozner a year ago. He put me on the Miami Mediterranean diet. I've been on it ever since, have lost twenty-eight pounds, and kept it off. I enjoy eating this way, and I find the diet quite easy to adhere to. I haven't just lost weight, I also have much more energy, and feel healthier and stronger. I eat a wide variety of delicious, healthy foods and I exercise daily by walking. Best of all, with this change in lifestyle and diet, I feel that I will live a longer and healthier life.

Why Choose the Miami Mediterranean Diet Instead?

The Miami Mediterranean diet—as a well-balanced diet including healthy fats and complex carbohydrates—offers the best alternative if you're looking to lose weight without sacrificing your health. There's a reason the Mediterranean diet has been around for thousands of years! By pairing the Miami Mediterranean diet with increased exercise and lowered stress, you can not just lose weight, but lower your cholesterol, blood sugar, and blood pressure—and as you've already seen, that's just the beginning of the benefits.

The Secret to Weight Loss

The secret to weight loss is simple: burn more calories than you consume. Americans consume too many calories! We eat large meals and then snack in the evening while we sit and watch TV. This excessive caloric intake combined with our sedentary lifestyle is the reason why obesity is a major public health threat.

We must learn to eat smart. First, we need to limit the portions of food we eat. Over the years, restaurant portions and packaged food portions have increased in size. The average bagel now weighs four to five ounces (equal to four or five slices of bread), cookies are the size of saucers, and an order of pasta in a restaurant would once have fed a family of four. To determine what an "average" serving of a packaged food is, check the nutrition label. You'll probably be surprised to learn that the "single" packaged food portion you assumed was for one is actually intended for two or more. You don't need to weigh and measure foods, but use common sense, and learn to eyeball correct portions. For instance, a medium-sized orange is about the size of a tennis ball, and a three-ounce piece of meat is the size and thickness of a deck of cards.

Second, we need to burn more calories by being physically active—there's no other way to do it!

Third, we must replace processed food, refined sugar, trans fats, and saturated fats with healthier, lower-calorie whole foods—as in the Miami Mediterranean diet.

People who live in the Mediterranean region and follow a Mediterranean diet and lifestyle are leaner than their American counterparts for a number of reasons:

- Exercise is a part of everyday life.
- Consumption of food with high fiber content, like fruits, vegetables, beans, nuts, and whole grains, leads to high satiety: a feeling of being full.
- Trans fats, which are associated with weight gain and obesity, are avoided, whereas healthy fats, such as monounsaturated fat and

omega-3 fat, are encouraged. Fat consumption, in the form of olive oil, nuts, and fish, also leads to satiety.

- Consumption of complex rather than simple carbohydrates, and avoidance of the refined sugars linked with obesity, makes the eater feel full longer.
- Food is not "super-sized" in Mediterranean countries like it is in America. It is the quality of food, not the quantity of food, that makes a good meal!

Lower Your Cholesterol—The Natural Way

In addition to weight loss, one of the chief benefits of the Miami Mediterranean diet and lifestyle is its impact on cholesterol. The Mediterranean diet has been shown to lower the bad (LDL) cholesterol, raise the good (HDL) cholesterol, and lower triglycerides. I have had many patients reduce or eliminate their cholesterol-lowering medications after several months on the Miami Mediterranean diet (but remember, any decision to adjust your medications should be made by your personal treating physician). This improvement in cholesterol helps explain the cardiovascular benefit of following a Mediterranean diet: it decreases the build-up of fatty deposits in artery walls.

The top foods responsible for the favorable impact on cholesterol are listed below—you may recognize many of them as the key nutritional components of the Mediterranean diet!

- Fruits and vegetables
- Whole grains (bread, cereal, etc.)
- Olive oil
- Nuts (especially almonds)
- Beans
- Soy protein
- Coldwater fish (and other foods rich in omega-3 fats)
- Red wine
- Cinnamon

There's a reason so many plants and plant products are included on this list. Whereas cholesterol is derived from animals, when we eat fruits, vegetables, and grains, we ingest plant sterols (or phytosterols), the plant equivalent. Plant sterols are beneficial because they interfere with the intestinal absorption of cholesterol, thereby lowering cholesterol levels. Certain vegetable spreads found in the grocery store also contain plant sterols, and can lower cholesterol and benefit long-term health, especially when used to replace butter or margarine.

In addition, exercise, an integral part of a Miami Mediterranean lifestyle, raises good (HDL) cholesterol, lowers triglycerides, and makes bad (LDL) cholesterol particles larger and less likely to cause heart attack and stroke.

Lower Your Blood Pressure with Diet and Lifestyle

Blood pressure is the term used to refer to the force of the blood against the artery walls, and it is measured in two numbers: systolic and diastolic. Systolic pressure is the level of force as the heart beats, and diastolic pressure is the level of force as the heart relaxes between beats. We used to think that only diastolic pressure was important, but both numbers matter in all individuals. Elevated systolic pressure is a key indicator of your risk for stroke, especially in the elderly population. Left uncontrolled, high blood pressure can also result in kidney disease, vascular disease, and increased risk of heart attack.

What is a normal reading? It used to be less than 140/90 millimeters of mercury (mmHg), with 120/80mm Hg being ideal. But according to recent changes in the guidelines, less than 120/80 mmHg is now considered optimal. The range between 120/80 mmHg and 140/90 mmHg is now called pre-hypertension. This guideline change means more people are now considered hypertensive or pre-hypertensive.

It is healthy for your blood pressure to fluctuate during the day due to physical activities or stressful stimuli, as it should return to normal as your body adjusts to the situation. But if it does not, it becomes a chronic condition called hypertension (elevated blood pressure). The condition is unfortunately common, affecting more than 50 million Americans.

While there is a lifestyle component to hypertension, the most common cause is aging. As we age, blood vessels lose their elasticity, or the ability to expand and contract. When the heart contracts and then relaxes, this reduced elasticity may lead to a rise in systolic pressure and a decrease in diastolic pressure.

Another common cause is heredity predisposition, as hypertension has a neurohormonal component that is under genetic control. People with a strong family history of hypertension are at higher risk of developing hypertension later in life compared to someone with no family history of the condition.

Hypertension caused by certain treatable conditions is called secondary hypertension. Reversible nutritional causes are surprisingly common. I always ask patients who show signs of hypertension if they eat licorice, as it contains glycyrrhizin, a substance that may cause sodium retention and thus can lead to hypertension. Excessive salt, alcohol, and caffeine can also increase blood pressure, so it is prudent to decrease or eliminate their consumption.

Other secondary causes of hypertension can be reversible through surgery. These include constriction or coarctation of the aorta, adrenal gland tumor (pheochromocytoma), or a blocked renal artery. People who snore might have obstructive sleep apnea, a cause of hypertension that has several treatment options.

Looking at the possible causes of hypertension, you can see that even someone who is leading the right lifestyle could still have a problem. This is why a complete evaluation by your personal physician is necessary: diagnosing and eliminating any secondary causes can significantly reduce or eliminate hypertension.

If you have no secondary causes, however, you should follow appropriate lifestyle changes, even if you also need medications (see the appendix for a list of common medications and what they do). I recommend a four-part program for all my patients with high blood pressure. The first three components, you'll notice, are also the cornerstones of the Miami Mediterranean diet and lifestyle: good nutrition, exercise, and stress management. The fourth, when applicable, is smoking cessation.

Nutrition

Many foods contain nutrients derived from plants (phytonutrients) that help lower blood pressure, so it makes sense to eat a diet rich in such foods. As it happens, those foods are beneficial for weight control, which can also help to reduce blood pressure. The Miami Mediterranean diet emphasizes the importance of eating heart-healthy fruits and vegetables, whole grains, olive oil, coldwater fish, low-fat dairy products, red wine, nuts, and beans—foods that can lower blood pressure. What the Miami Mediterranean diet does not contain is also important: it is low in saturated fat, has no trans fat, and is low in sodium—all factors that can lower blood pressure.

We have long seen the evidence that a Mediterranean diet supports cardiovascular health and can lower blood pressure, and science has backed this theory. Fruits, vegetables, and nuts provide potassium, calcium, and magnesium for lowering blood pressure. Extra-virgin olive oil supports healthy blood pressure by causing blood vessels to dilate. Red wine in moderation (one 5-ounce glass per day for women, and two for men) and red or purple grape juice may help relax arteries, which can lower blood pressure. Numerous studies have documented the blood pressure–regulating benefits of fresh garlic, abundant in a Mediterranean diet. And fish is rich in omega-3 fatty acids, which are beneficial for numerous disease states, including hypertension.

Exercise

We exercise far too little, which is unfortunate, since exercise lowers blood pressure in a couple of ways. One way is by supporting weight loss, particularly the reduction of abdominal fat. Fat in this area is associated with elevated levels of a protein called angiotensinogen, which can lead to hypertension. Exercise also strengthens the heart and makes the cardiovascular system more efficient by relaxing and dilating blood vessels. And if you exercise rather than raiding the refrigerator as an outlet for stress, you can both eliminate emotional eating and maintain a healthy weight.

Stress Management

Stress releases catecholamines, chemicals that prepare the body for physical activity and can therefore increase blood pressure. There is ample evidence that managing and reducing stress can significantly lower the risk of hypertension. We know this from the works of Dr. Herbert Benson of Harvard University, who popularized a stress-reduction technique in his book *The Relaxation Response*, and from cardiologist Dr. Robert S. Eliot, who coined the phrase "the hot reactor" for his patients who had an exaggerated rise in heart rate or blood pressure in response to stimuli that would only cause a small reaction in an average person.

There are many stress-reduction techniques to choose from: transcendental meditation, self-hypnosis, breathing techniques, Benson's relaxation response, yoga, prayer, and deep muscle relaxation. Find something that works for you and that you enjoy. Your exercise program may also reduce stress and make you better able to handle the stress you do encounter. Whatever method you choose, just stick with it!

Smoking Cessation

A word about smoking: Quit! This is a no-brainer. Cigarette smoking increases the risk of developing heart disease for a variety of reasons. The nicotine causes arteries to constrict, and the carbon monoxide from cigarette smoke decreases the amount of oxygenated blood reaching the heart muscle. No amount of smoking is safe, and it is counterproductive to an otherwise healthy lifestyle. There are many methods to help you quit, including nicotine patches or gum, acupuncture, and hypnosis, to name a few. Several new medications are also available to help "kick the habit." If you are unable to quit on your own, discuss smoking cessation with your doctor—don't let your good health go up in smoke!

Putting the Pieces Together

There are many important components to the Miami Mediterranean diet, and although each component is responsible for conferring a certain degree of health, it is the combination of all of the components that makes the Miami Mediterranean diet so beneficial. The better you understand how each component contributes to your overall health, however, the better you'll be at understanding how everything works together.

This section goes more in depth on a few of the most important aspects of the Miami Mediterranean diet. As a result, you'll be more capable than ever of making the best food choices for your health.

Fat: The Good, the Bad, and the Ugly

There are three types of fat in our diet: unsaturated fat, saturated fat, and trans fat...or the good, the bad, and the ugly.

The Good

Unsaturated fats, including polyunsaturated fats and monounsaturated fats, are good fats. Omega-3 and omega-6 fatty acids are polyunsaturated fats. Omega-3, which comes from oily fish, vegetables, and nuts, is cardioprotective (decreases the risk of heart disease). Monosaturated fat, from nuts, seeds, and olive oil, is also cardioprotective, thought to be beneficial since it has a positive impact on our cholesterol ratio and helps to decrease inflammation. Vegetable oils (which include various amounts of both mono- and polyunsaturated fat) like soybean, sunflower, and corn oils, are neutral, meaning they have no effect, either good or bad, on heart health.

The Bad

Saturated fats, which raise the bad (LDL) cholesterol and increase the risk of heart disease and cancer, are bad fats. They're found in animal products, such as red meat, butter, milk, cheese, and lard, as well as tropical oils, like coconut and palm oils.

The Ugly

Then there are trans fatty acids, or trans fats. These fats are particularly harmful to our health, as they raise the bad (LDL) cholesterol, lower the good (HDL) cholesterol, increase inflammation, and make blood more likely to form clots. Trans fat consumption has been linked to heart disease, cancer, and diabetes.

Trans fats are found in foods such as margarine, French fries, potato chips, cookies, crackers, baked goods, and frozen foods. Trans fats don't occur naturally. They're manufactured by taking oils—mainly vegetable oils—and putting them through a process called hydrogenation, and were developed so that foods could last longer on the shelf without becoming rancid.

The biggest problem with the American diet is that we consume too much saturated fat and trans fat. In fact, certain countries have actually banned trans fat from their food supply! Until America does the same, the best course of action is to pay attention to nutrition labels, avoid food that contains trans fat or partially hydrogenated oil, and limit our consumption of saturated fat.

Omega-3 Deficiency: The Scurvy of Our Time

It has been suggested that up to 90% of Americans are omega-3 deficient. How can that be? Prior to the Industrial Revolution and the migration from the farm to the city, the vast majority of our food was grown locally. Our fruits and vegetables were good sources of omega-3 fat, and since cattle were free-roaming and grass-fed, they too consumed naturally occurring omega-3, which we took in when we ate beef. Today we live in a different world. Food is shipped from farms to grocery stores, and so requires the inclusion of preservatives. Our soil has been depleted of its nutrients, and cattle are sedentary grain-fed creatures, woefully deficient in omega-3.

Why should this matter? The ratio of omega-3 to omega-6 in our body is important to health maintenance: omega-3 fat is anti-inflammatory, whereas omega-6 fat is pro-inflammatory. The omega-6/omega-3 ratio should be 1/1; however, due to the decrease in omega-3 intake and an increase in omega-6 intake (especially via corn oil and red meat), the omega-6/omega-3 ratio in the average American is somewhere between 10/1 to 20/1. This imbalance is associated with an increase in:

- Acne
- Allergies
- Arthritis
- Asthma
- Cancer
- Depression
- Diabetes
- Disorder of the heart rhythm
- Heart disease
- Hypertension
- Inflammatory bowel disease
- Sudden cardiac death

The Miami Mediterranean diet alters this ratio by providing your body with ample amounts of omega-3 fat and limiting the amount of omega-6 fat you consume.

Carbohydrates: Simple and Complex

Carbohydrates are a source of energy and nutrition that is essential to good health. Simple carbohydrates like candy and soda are sugars, which are quickly absorbed into our bloodstream and provide an immediate source of energy. Complex carbohydrates like whole grain bread and cereal, oatmeal, and apples (also known as polysaccharides or starches) are made of long strands of sugars and are broken down and metabolized more slowly, providing the body with energy over a longer period of time. Consequently, they are more filling and help curb appetite.

A good way to think of this is in terms of foods' glycemic index. The glycemic index is a ranking of various foods based on the speed at which those foods are able to increase blood sugar or glucose compared to white bread, which was given an arbitrary glycemic index of 100. Foods which increase blood sugar faster than white bread have a glycemic index greater than 100; foods which increase blood sugar slower than white bread are assigned a glycemic index less than 100. Carbohydrates with more fiber and less sugar have glycemic indexes less than 100, meaning that they will leave you feeling full longer. Compared to simple carbohydrates, complex carbohydrates with low glycemic indexes improve blood glucose levels and decrease your likelihood of developing diabetes and heart disease. (Fortunately, you don't need to memorize the glycemic index of food; simply by following the Miami Mediterranean diet, you will be consuming heart-healthy non-processed food with a low glycemic index.)

Foods to Avoid: The Hidden Danger of High Fructose Corn Syrup

It's smart to avoid table sugar, but there's an even more sinister sweetener lurking on your supermarket shelves: high fructose corn syrup. This sweetener is a favorite of the food industry since it is sweeter than ordinary table sugar, is inexpensive, and prolongs the shelf-life of food. It is found in many beverages and foods, including soft drinks, sports drinks, packaged cookies, and other baked goods. Since its introduction in 1970, the amount of high fructose corn syrup in our food has steadily increased; currently the average American consumes 73.5 pounds of this sweetener each year. Our obesity rate also jumped from 15% to 30% during the same period, which many nutritionists believe is not a coincidence.

The real danger posed by high fructose corn syrup, however, is the metabolic havoc it causes. In contrast to ordinary sugar, high fructose corn syrup is not utilized by the muscles as an energy source. Instead, it goes directly to the liver and leads to an increase in triglyceride production.

Water: The Fountain of Youth

It is essential to consume an adequate amount of water each day: at least six to eight glasses, or 48 ounces. When we don't drink enough water we become dehydrated. This causes our blood to become thicker and more likely to clot, which can result in a sudden heart attack or stroke. People who live in tropical climates need to drink even more water, because they lose fluid through perspiration.

Not only is drinking water throughout the day a healthful thing to do, it can also help you lose weight. Sometimes it's difficult to distinguish whether you are hungry or thirsty. If you drink a glass of water, and then wait twenty to thirty minutes before eating, you may find that your hunger has been eliminated, or at least diminished. Furthermore, water is important to your body's ability to function properly, gives your skin a healthy glow, and improves muscle tone. Refreshing water indeed is a fountain of youth.

But water is not the only drink available to us. What about our other options?

Fruit and Vegetable Juices

Although higher in calories than water, fruit juice, enjoyed in moderation, also has its place in the Miami Mediterranean diet. Fruit juice doesn't replace the need to eat whole fruit, which has fiber and makes you feel full, but can still be a refreshing source of nutrients and disease-fighting antioxidants.

Which fruit juice to choose? Drinking a wide variety of juices can bring a host of disease-fighting vitamins, minerals, and antioxidants to the table. Purple grape juice and cranberry juice are particularly good sources of antioxidants. Orange juice has vitamin C, potassium, and folic acid. Grapefruit juice also has vitamin C and potassium, but also contains a chemical that can interfere with the metabolism or breakdown of certain medications (check with your doctor or pharmacist if you take any medications).

Pomegranate juice is also a great choice. The pomegranate's popularity is on the rise lately, thanks mostly to the growing interest in its health benefits. Like many other fruit juices, this sweet-and-tangy drink is loaded with a combination of antioxidants for a particularly potent effect.

Research studies have found that pomegranate juice helps lower blood pressure, reduce the buildup of atherosclerotic plaque, and preserve nitric oxide, key in keeping the coronary arteries healthy. Pomegranate juice is also a great source of vitamin C and potassium, and contains less sugar than some other fruit juices. (Don't let the enthusiasm for pomegranate juice discourage you from trying the fruit itself, though; it's perfect for eating and cooking.)

Vegetable juices offer many of the same benefits as their fruity counterparts. Tomato juice and V-8, for example, are great low-calorie sources of vitamins and minerals. These juices contain a significant amount of sodium, however, which can lead to high blood pressure and fluid retention. Low-sodium tomato juice or V-8 is preferable—you can add potassium salt for taste if desired.

Finally, when it comes to fruit and vegetable juices, just don't go overboard—moderation is the key!

Fruit Drinks—Caution!

Many people consume fruit drinks thinking that they are healthy. Beware—these drinks are often nothing more than flavored sugar water, and have little to no nutritional value. Also, these beverages are often marketed to children and can contribute to childhood obesity. Remember, whole fruit paired with a glass of good old-fashioned water is still your best nutritional bet!

Enjoy Your Morning Coffee, but Don't Forget Your Afternoon Tea!

Though drinking anything containing caffeine can worsen dehydration (because it has a diuretic effect that can lead to fluid loss), one or two cups of coffee a day is fine, as long as you avoid rich, blended coffee drinks. Don't let your love affair with coffee blind you from the possibility of enjoying a cup of tea, however. Both coffee and tea can be enjoyed hot or iced, and both also contain antioxidants and chemicals that have been found to reduce the risk of diabetes, gallstones, and kidney stones. But it is tea that contains substances that help reduce the risk of heart disease and cancer.

Green tea, for instance, is rich in catechin polyphenols such as ECGC, a potent antioxidant which has been shown to be twice as powerful as resveratrol (another powerful antioxidant found in red wine). In addition,

ECGC lowers bad (LDL) cholesterol, inhibits blood clot formation, and inhibits the growth of cancer cells. Finally, green tea has been shown to aid in weight loss and also help prevent dental plaque.

Does the color of the tea matter? Both black tea and green tea come from the same source: the white-flowered *Camellia sinensis* plant, which is loaded with antioxidants and gives tea its cardiovascular benefits. Green tea may have an edge because it's made from young tea leaves, providing more antioxidant power and boosting its health benefits. But if you prefer black tea, or it's the type you have handy, don't be dissuaded from enjoying it, because it's a healthy brew as well. The same goes for white tea.

To release tea's strongest health benefits, brew it yourself, using either the leaves or a tea bag, and let it steep in the cup for three to five minutes (though different color teas may require different brewing times; check the packaging). Bear in mind that although you may enjoy herbal teas, pure tea provides more antioxidant punch.

Wine, Whiskey, or Beer?

It used to be said that wine was preferable to whiskey or beer for heart health. Clinical studies, however, have shown that all forms of alcohol are beneficial for cardiovascular disease prevention—providing they are consumed in moderation! Moderation is defined as one drink a day for a woman and two drinks a day for a man (one drink: 5 ounces of wine; 1.5 ounces of whiskey; 12 ounces of beer). Nevertheless, several studies have suggested that red wine (rich in the antioxidant resveratrol) does have additional health benefits beyond beer or whiskey. As the debate continues regarding the optimal form of alcohol, however, the following remains clear:

- Alcohol, in any form, is not encouraged for cardiovascular disease prevention in those who already abstain from drinking—there are better ways to prevent heart disease (such as a healthy lifestyle and medical therapy if required).
- There is a dark side to alcohol consumption, especially when consumed in excess (addiction, liver disease, increased incidence of certain cancers, cardiomyopathy and heart rhythm disorders, accidents—especially automobile accidents, etc.).
- If you choose to consume alcohol, do so in moderation!

Wine consumption has been enjoyed since antiquity in the Mediterranean regions of the world. Nevertheless, it was never consumed in isolation—it was enjoyed with delicious food and shared among family and friends.

Milk: Friend or Foe?

One of our most prevalent American myths is the health benefit of drinking three or more glasses of whole milk per day. Besides increasing cholesterol due to its saturated fat content, whole milk has been a big contributor to the obesity epidemic in America and developed nations worldwide. Note that three 8-ounce glasses of milk a day deliver 450 calories and 15 grams of saturated fat. In addition, the hormones cows are given to increase their milk production, as well as the antibiotics they're fed to prevent infection, have also been found in blood samples of milk drinkers.

Regular milk consumption may increase the risk of:

- Diabetes
- GI disturbances (due to lactose intolerance)
- Heart disease
- Multiple sclerosis
- Ovarian cancer
- Prostate cancer

If you must consume milk, enjoying fat-free or skim milk in moderation makes more sense. Likewise, choose low-fat or fat-free cheese, select low-fat or fat-free yogurt, and switch from butter and margarine to olive oil or a trans fat–free vegetable spread for your other dairy needs. Finally, for all you ice cream junkies out there, consider fat-free ice milk or a fresh fruit sorbet—your heart will thank you!

Don't Lose Your Whey

Dairy isn't all bad, however. Whey, once considered a waste byproduct of cheese manufacturing, is now prized as a high-quality, protein-packed snack that is low in fat and easily digested.

Known as a "fast" protein, whey provides a host of health benefits beyond the speed at which it's absorbed. Amino acids, the body's "building blocks," are necessary for the growth and repair of tissue, and whey's specific combination of these substances helps stabilize blood sugar and boosts the immune system. When it comes to heart health, whey has been found to benefit cholesterol by raising good (HDL) cholesterol and lowering triglycerides. Whey protein also promotes the growth of lean muscle and helps burn abdominal fat.

Regular dairy products contain lactose, which is milk sugar, but whey is lactose-free and a good choice for people who are lactose intolerant. Whey protein is generally safe; however, it should be consumed in moderation, as excessive protein consumption can lead to kidney impairment. For most people, a whey protein smoothie or shake as a substitute meal or snack several times a week, in addition to a healthy diet and lifestyle, is perfectly acceptable; however, be sure to discuss this with your doctor.

Free Radicals: The Result of a Toxic American Diet and Lifestyle

If you cut an apple in half and let it sit on your countertop, it turns brown in a matter of minutes. A metal pipe left outside in the rain and elements begins to rust in due time. This process is called oxidation—and it happens in our bodies, too.

Free radicals are a key part of this. Free radicals are unstable atoms continuously produced as a byproduct of oxygen, as oxygen is used for fuel in the human body. In a stable atom, the nucleus is surrounded by a cloud of paired electrons. Free radicals, in contrast, are atoms that contain an odd number of electrons, meaning that one pair is missing an electron. Because of this, free radicals are highly unstable and very reactive. As free radicals come into contact with other, normal atoms, they steal their electrons to replace the missing one, creating new free radicals and starting an ongoing chain reaction. This is the same process of oxidation that makes apples turn brown and metal rust. In the human body, it causes tissue damage at the cellular level, affecting DNA, the cell mitochondria, and the cell membrane, and eventually causing cell death. This, in turn, leads to both aging and disease. In addition, free radical production can lead to the buildup of fatty deposits in the artery wall (atherosclerosis), as well as blood clot formation and coronary artery spasm.

Today, the human body is exposed to many more external environmental toxins than in the past. These toxins act as catalysts, multiplying the free radical chain reaction in our bodies by several thousand, perhaps even several million.

Examples of toxins that lead to free radical formation:

- Pollutants in our air (such as carbon monoxide from cigarette smoke and automobile exhaust)
- Ultraviolet rays from the sun
- Pesticides
- Ionizing radiation from X-rays and procedures like CAT scans
- Radiation exposure from television and computer screens
- Excess alcohol consumption
- Processed foods
- Trans fats

It has also been shown that consuming a high-fat diet leads to elevated levels of free radicals called lipid peroxides (free radicals formed from fat); a low-fat diet, on the other hand, reduces the production of lipid peroxides.

Where Do Antioxidants Come From, and How Do They Work?

The natural internal production of free radicals is an inevitable byproduct of life, and our body has evolved a natural array of antioxidant nutrients to help rein free radicals in, keeping them from doing extensive damage. However, we are adding thousands more free radicals into our bodies through environmental toxins, and our body isn't equipped to handle them alone. That's why it's so important to take in additional antioxidants in the form of fruits and vegetables. If we don't get enough antioxidants, our bodies are in danger.

Antioxidants are the body's defense system—they combat and quench the biochemical fires that result from free radical formation. In fact, antioxidants can deactivate free radicals before extensive damage can been done. Antioxidants are capable of donating an electron to free radicals, thereby neutralizing them and ending the electron-stealing chain reaction that would otherwise take place. The antioxidants themselves do not become free radicals because they are stable even when they are missing an electron.

Foods to Avoid: My Beef with Red Meat

Americans eat too much red meat—they have bacon or sausage for breakfast, a hamburger or hot dog for lunch, steak for dinner, and then wake up and do it all over again. This is not healthy!

Excessive consumption of red meat has been linked to:

- Cancer (including colorectal cancer, breast cancer, prostate cancer, and pancreatic cancer)
- Diabetes
- Elevated cholesterol
- Heart disease
- Hypertension
- Chronic inflammation

In addition, red meat may contain:

- Bacteria
- Heterocyclic amines (which have been linked to cancer)
- Hormones
- PCBs (which are toxic)
- Protein prions (which have been linked to bovine spongiform encephalopathy, also known as mad cow disease)
- Viruses

Americans and other Western societies should follow the example set by people living in the Mediterranean: if you consume meat, do so less frequently (weekly or monthly, not daily), and when you do, utilize lean cuts of meat. Meat is often used as flavoring in a Mediterranean meal rather than the meal itself.

So enjoy your occasional meat dish—just not to excess!

The principal micronutrient (or vitamin) antioxidants are vitamin E, vitamin C, and beta-carotene. But since our bodies do not manufacture these micronutrients, they must be supplied externally through the food we eat. The best way to protect ourselves from the ravages of oxidation and free radicals is nutrition. Consumption of a wide variety of fruits and vegetables provides thousands of antioxidants and phytonutrients that work in concert with one another to fight disease.

It is recommended that you eat at least five to nine servings of fruits and vegetables per day. I recommend that you select a wide variety of colors when choosing those fruits and vegetables, since this ensures you'll be consuming lots of different phytonutrients and antioxidants. For example:

- Oranges provide vitamin C
- Tomatoes provide lycopene
- Carrots provide beta-carotene
- Blueberries provide anthocyanins
- Spinach provides lutein and zeaxanthin
- Purple grapes provide resveratrol

In addition to fruits and vegetables, whole grains, nuts, beans, fish, and other foods common to a Mediterranean diet help to reduce free radical damage in our bodies. They contain a variety of different antioxidants such as selenium, zinc, and other minerals and essential amino acids. All of these antioxidants work in different areas of cells to control and neutralize free radicals and prevent disease. It is the full spectrum of antioxidants working together with one another that promotes good health. And all of the thousands of antioxidants that you need can be obtained by eating a healthy diet.

What About Vitamins?

The processing of food unfortunately removes many of the vitamins, phytochemicals, and micronutrients that we need for our long-term health. The best way to take in these vitamins and nutrients is by eating non-processed whole foods. But might vitamins be an acceptable substitute?

Despite our best efforts, we are unable to duplicate what Mother Nature provides with a healthy diet by simply taking vitamin pills. Taking a few vitamins in high doses to stay healthy just doesn't work. Clinical trials have failed to show any benefit to taking large doses of select vitamins; in fact, vitamins can actually be detrimental to our health if taken in large doses. Vitamin A and niacin, for example, can be toxic in large amounts. We need the whole package, thousands of antioxidant vitamins and minerals, to stay healthy. A daily multivitamin can be beneficial as an "insurance policy" against gaps in nutrition, but only provided it is taken *in addition* to a healthy diet—not in place of it!

Fish oil capsules, to increase omega-3 intake, may be an exception. Several large clinical trials have demonstrated the value of consuming an adequate amount of fish, but in one large Italian study, more than 10,000 men and women with preexisting heart disease were given fish oil or a placebo, and those taking fish oil capsules had a 45% reduction in their risk of sudden cardiac death. Other clinical trials have also demonstrated cardiovascular benefit from fish oil. A Japanese study demonstrated that the addition of fish oil to statin medication in patients with elevated cholesterol resulted in a reduced risk of heart attacks and death from heart disease as compared to patients who were placed on statins without fish oil.

So should you take omega-3 laden fish oil supplements? If your intake of coldwater fish is limited, it might be worth considering. But since high doses of fish oil may thin the blood, they should not be taken without medical supervision.

Cinnamon: The Spice of Life

Too often in America, we remove cinnamon from the cupboard only on special occasions, to flavor pumpkin pies for Thanksgiving or bake cookies during the Christmas holidays. No more! It's time to steal a secret that other countries like China and India know: that cinnamon not only flavors food, but offers health benefits as well.

Ground cinnamon is made from the bark of the cinnamon tree and it contains three types of essential oils (cinnamaldehyde, cinnamyl acetate, and cinnamyl alcohol) that provide it with health-boosting properties, as well as a wide range of other active substances. These oils have different beneficial effects: they act as an anti-coagulant, preventing blood from forming heart-attack-causing clots; they have anti-inflammatory properties; and they enhance the ability of diabetics to metabolize sugar. There's even some research indicating the smell of cinnamon can help improve brain activity.

And you don't have to down copious amounts of cinnamon to reap its benefits; research shows that less than a half-teaspoon of cinnamon a day lowers blood glucose levels and improves the cholesterol balance in people at high risk for diabetes and coronary heart disease.

Cinnamon tastes great, so it's also an inexpensive, easy way to brighten up a vast variety of recipes. Use cinnamon to spice up hot beverages, like tea or apple cider, or sprinkle it on top of sugar-free cocoa. Dust it on squash or carrots, or swirl it into yogurt and add a dash of honey for a quick dessert. Just leaf through this book and you'll find many recipes in the Miami Mediterranean diet that utilize this versatile and healthful spice. But perhaps the best tip of all is to take that container of cinnamon down from the shelf, transfer its contents to a shaker, and leave it on the kitchen table. That way, you'll keep it on hand, and use it often.

The Miami Mediterranean "Salt Shaker"

Forget table salt—it contains sodium, which increases your risk of high blood pressure, stroke, and heart attack. Instead, take a salt shaker and fill it with equal parts potassium salt, garlic powder, onion powder, and black pepper. Your heart will thank you!

Dark Chocolate: It Tastes Too Good to Be Healthy!

Not everything that tastes good is bad for you. Take chocolate!

Chocolate can be enjoyed on the Miami Mediterranean diet, as long as it is dark chocolate. Chocolate is made from cocoa beans, which are one of the richest sources of beneficial antioxidants, especially flavanols. Flavanols help lower blood pressure, balance cholesterol, and maintain a favorable blood glucose level. But it is flavanols that give chocolate a bitter taste, so confectioners remove them and then add refined sugar and fat. *Voilà*! The result is unhealthy milk chocolate.

Dark chocolate, on the other hand, is the darling of chocolate connoisseurs, who prefer its less sweet, more interesting taste. And thanks to its flavanols, dark chocolate also makes the grade for inclusion in the Miami Mediterranean diet, as long as it's enjoyed in moderation. Confectionary companies are catching on and touting dark chocolate's health merits. But always read the nutrition label, and choose dark chocolates that are lowest in saturated fat and sugar, have no trans fats, and contain at least 70% cocoa flavanols.

Remember, no matter how it's touted, dark chocolate still has plenty of calories, so enjoy it in moderation and, when you do indulge, don't gobble it up. Instead, savor a piece or two, perhaps with a glass of red wine, as a delightful ending to a Miami Mediterranean meal.

There Is No Need to Desert the Dessert

You don't need to be deprived; you can enjoy scrumptious desserts while on the Miami Mediterranean diet. In this book you will find a variety of new and exciting desserts that will satisfy even the most discriminating palate.

The problem with most traditional American desserts is their use of high fructose corn syrup, saturated fats, and trans fats— all unhealthy ingredients that have a high calorie content. Not so for the desserts found in the second half of this book. These desserts are not only delicious but have no trans fats, are very low in saturated fat content, and do not contain high fructose corn syrup. There's even a 5-calorie cookie!

It's Your Choice!

You've seen the dangers of the American diet—and you've seen the benefits of the alternative. In particular, you've seen the threat that cardiovascular disease poses. Now you have to make a choice.

There are two different pathways that you can travel in the war against cardiovascular disease. The first pathway is called the dead-end road. Those who travel down the dead-end road refuse to learn about cardiovascular disease prevention. Their attitude is, "I'll wait until I have chest pain and then I'll worry about it." They frequently criticize people who take medications, saying, "The medications have adverse side effects which can cause serious problems and I simply won't take them." They refuse to exercise or eat a heart-healthy diet. The dead-end road eventually leads to the number one cause of death in the United States and most developed countries in the world—cardiovascular disease.

The second pathway is called progress road. People who travel down progress road refuse to succumb to cardiovascular disease without a fight. They understand the basic principles of cardiovascular disease prevention. They maintain a heart-healthy diet and exercise on a regular basis. They have appropriate blood tests to screen for cardiovascular disease, and they understand the current guidelines for cholesterol and triglyceride management. If they have an elevated cholesterol or triglyceride level, they seek out appropriate medical attention so they can receive proper treatment. Those who travel down the progress road have a much lower likelihood of being hospitalized with a heart attack or undergoing expensive and risky procedures such as bypass surgery or stent placement. Progress road ultimately leads to cardiovascular health!

Let us not underestimate our enemy. Cardiovascular disease claims more lives than any other disease: every thirty seconds someone will die from a heart attack in America. Certainly if we were fighting an external enemy this formidable, we would do whatever it took to win the war.

If you're ready to fight, read on. The next section will provide you with all the information you need to begin the Miami Mediterranean diet, and start you on a journey of lifelong health.

Robert's Story

I was a forty-eight-year-old male executive who often worked a sixty-hour week and played tennis occasionally, whenever I could fit it into my hectic schedule. I was divorced and tended to eat out, often just grabbing two double cheeseburgers with bacon and super-sized fries at the nearest fast food restaurant. I also ate potato chips for snacks. I seldom saw a doctor, except for an occasional bad cold. Other than being fifteen pounds overweight, I considered myself to be in fairly good health. When I was a young boy my parents always encouraged me to eat foods high in protein and fat because they thought those foods would make me strong and healthy. Except for in my ice cream or on my pizza, I seldom consumed either fruit or vegetables. Also, fish was just not part of my vocabulary.

One Sunday afternoon about six months ago, I was playing a grueling game of tennis when I suddenly developed tightness in my chest. It was severe enough to cause me to stop and take notice. Two days later I saw a doctor, who led me to a heart evaluation by a cardiologist. I underwent a heart catheterization and a stent was placed in one of my coronary arteries. While I was hospitalized, I heard about Dr. Ozner from the nurses taking care of me. He had just given a lecture on heart disease prevention and they were all buzzing about his approach of preventive care. It was then that I decided to make an appointment to see him.

Dr. Ozner educated me about cardiovascular health and the

role that diet, exercise, and stress management play in maintaining good health. He said that I could significantly reduce my likelihood of having a heart attack if I changed my current lifestyle and eating habits. He gave me a copy of his book, *The Miami Mediterranean Diet*. After reading the book, it became clear to me that a diet of high protein and saturated fat actually contributed to my chances of dying from a heart attack. So I tried the Miami Mediterranean diet, and realized it was not only a healthy and nutritious way to eat, but also a delicious one! Although I still take medications, I have improved my diet, and I exercise on a regular basis. I am confident that these measures will decrease my chances of having a heart attack or dying prematurely from heart disease.

PART TWO

RECIPES

A 14-Day Menu Plan

The Miami Mediterranean diet is not a quick weight-loss diet plan but rather a healthy nutritional plan that will help you reach and maintain your optimal weight, and this sample 14-day menu plan will help get you started.

You may substitute any Mediterranean recipe for those listed in the 14-day menu plan. In addition, you are encouraged to eat a wide variety of fruits and vegetables of many different colors. All of the recipes in this book are made from fresh, healthy, non-processed foods. The fat content included in these recipes is mainly unsaturated fat (especially monounsaturated fat and omega-3 fat), with limited saturated fat and no trans fat. Remember to exercise daily and adjust your portion size to achieve ideal body weight.

Bon appetit!

DAY 1

BREAKFAST

4 ounces vegetable or fruit juice
1 slice whole wheat toast with extra-virgin olive oil or 1 teaspoon vegetable
  spread (trans fat–free canola/olive oil spread)
1 teaspoon jam
½ cup plain low-fat yogurt (sweetened with non-caloric sweetener if desired)
½ cup blueberries or strawberries
8 ounces water
Coffee or tea (soy or non-fat milk, trans fat–free coffee creamer, and non-
  caloric sweetener if desired)

- APPROX. 239 CALORIES

OPTIONAL MIDMORNING SNACK

10–20 almonds or walnuts
8 ounces water or non-caloric beverage

LUNCH

Chickpea Pita Pocket (page 276)
1 medium apple, sliced and drizzled with honey
8 ounces water or non-caloric beverage

- APPROX. 319 CALORIES

OPTIONAL MIDDAY SNACK

10–20 almonds or walnuts
8 ounces water or non-caloric beverage

DINNER

1 jumbo clove Roasted Garlic (page 335)
½ (6-inch) whole wheat pita loaf, split open, sprayed with olive oil and herb
  seasonings of choice, and toasted in the microwave or oven until crispy
Goat Cheese Stuffed Tomato (page 74)
Linguine and Mixed Seafood (page 178)
Fresh vegetable of choice (flavor with olive oil or vegetable spread as desired)
Drunken Apricots (page 307)

8 ounces water

1 or 2 (4-ounce) glasses of red wine or purple grape juice

Coffee or tea (soy milk or non-fat, trans fat–free coffee creamer and non-caloric sweetener if desired)

• APPROX. 761 CALORIES

OPTIONAL EVENING SNACK

1 apple or orange

8 ounces water

DAY 2

BREAKFAST

4 ounces vegetable or fruit juice

½ cup egg whites with diced onions, tomato, and green bell peppers cooked into an omelet

1 slice whole wheat toast with extra-virgin olive oil or 1 teaspoon vegetable spread (trans fat–free canola/olive oil spread)

1 teaspoon fruit jam

½ small banana

8 ounces water

Coffee or tea (soy or non-fat milk, trans fat–free coffee creamer, and non-caloric sweetener if desired)

• APPROX. 230 CALORIES

OPTIONAL MIDMORNING SNACK

10–20 almonds or walnuts

8 ounces water or non-caloric beverage

LUNCH

Greek Olive and Feta Cheese Pasta Salad (page 73)

½ (6-inch) whole wheat pita loaf, toasted if desired

⅛-inch fresh cantaloupe

8 ounces water or non-caloric beverage

• APPROX. 354 CALORIES

OPTIONAL MIDDAY SNACK

1 apple
8 ounces water or non-caloric beverage

DINNER

1 jumbo clove Roasted Garlic (page 335)
½ (6-inch) whole wheat pita loaf, split open, sprayed with olive oil and herb
seasonings of choice, and toasted until crispy in the oven or microwave
6–8 marinated assorted olives
Grilled Citrus Salmon with Garlic Greens (page 157)
Grilled Eggplant (page 260)
Strawberries and Balsamic Syrup (page 305)
8 ounces water
1 or 2 (4-ounce) glasses of red wine or purple grape juice
Coffee or tea (soy or non-fat milk, trans fat–free coffee creamer, and non-
caloric sweetener if desired)

• APPROX. 653 CALORIES

OPTIONAL EVENING SNACK

1 apple or orange
8 ounces water

DAY 3

BREAKFAST

4 ounces vegetable or fruit juice
½ cup egg whites with diced onions, tomato, and green bell peppers
1 slice whole wheat toast with olive oil (extra-virgin) or 1 teaspoon vegetable
spread (trans fat–free canola/olive oil spread)
1 teaspoon fruit jam
1 medium fresh peach or 1 large plum
8 ounces water
Coffee or tea (soy or non-fat milk, trans fat–free coffee creamer, and non-
caloric sweetener if desired)

• APPROX. 230 CALORIES

OPTIONAL MIDMORNING SNACK

10–20 almonds or walnuts
8 ounces water or non-caloric beverage

LUNCH

Italian Minestrone Soup with Pesto (page 104)
1 slice whole grain crusty bread with extra-virgin olive oil
½ cup fresh raspberries
½ cup plain low-fat yogurt, sweetened with non-caloric sweetener if desired
8 ounces water or non-caloric beverage

- APPROX. 390 CALORIES

OPTIONAL MIDDAY SNACK

1 apple
8 ounces water or non-caloric beverage

DINNER

Simple Spanish Salad (page 90)
1 jumbo clove Roasted Garlic (page 335)
½ (6-inch) whole wheat pita loaf, split open, sprayed with olive oil and herb
seasonings of choice, and toasted until crispy in the oven or microwave
1 slice soft goat cheese
6–8 marinated mixed olives
Fresh vegetable of choice (flavor with olive oil or vegetable spread as desired)
Chicken Piccata (page 188)
Honeydew Sorbet (page 304)
8 ounces water
1 or 2 (4-ounce) glasses of red wine or purple grape juice
Coffee or tea (soy or non-fat milk, trans fat–free coffee creamer, and non-caloric sweetener if desired)

- APPROX. 725 CALORIES

OPTIONAL EVENING SNACK

2 Meringue Cookies (page 316)
Green tea or 8 ounces water

DAY 4

BREAKFAST

4 ounces vegetable or fruit juice
2 slices whole wheat toast
2 tablespoons fresh chunky peanut butter
2 teaspoons honey
½ ruby red grapefruit, sweetened with non-caloric sweetener if desired
8 ounces water
Coffee or tea (soy or non-fat milk, trans fat–free coffee creamer, and non-caloric sweetener if desired)

- APPROX. 385 CALORIES

OPTIONAL MIDMORNING SNACK

10–20 almonds or walnuts
8 ounces water or non-caloric beverage

LUNCH

Light Caesar Salad (page 85)
1 slice Pizza Margherita (page 123)
10–20 seedless grapes
8 ounces water or non-caloric beverage

- APPROX. 302 CALORIES

OPTIONAL MIDDAY SNACK

1 apple
8 ounces water or non-caloric beverage

DINNER

1 clove jumbo Roasted Garlic (page 335)
½ (6-inch) whole wheat pita loaf, split open, sprayed with extra-virgin olive oil and herb seasonings of choice, and toasted until crispy in the oven or microwave
Chilly Tomato Soup (page 103)
Fennel Salad (page 82)
Fresh vegetable of choice (flavor with olive oil or vegetable spread as desired)
Spicy Whole Wheat Capellini with Garlic (page 161)

8 ounces water
Sweet Plum Compote (page 297)
1 or 2 (4-ounce) glasses of red wine or purple grape juice
Coffee or tea (soy or non-fat milk, trans fat–free coffee creamer, and non-
  caloric sweetener if desired)

- approx. 786 calories

OPTIONAL EVENING SNACK

1 apple or orange
8 ounces water

DAY 5

BREAKFAST

4 ounces vegetable or fruit juice
1 slice whole wheat toast with extra-virgin olive oil or 1 teaspoon vegetable
  spread (trans fat–free canola/olive oil spread)
1 teaspoon fruit jam
½ cup plain low-fat yogurt, sweetened with non-caloric sweetener if desired
½ cup blueberries or strawberries
8 ounces water
Coffee or tea (soy or non-fat milk, trans fat–free coffee creamer, and non-
  caloric sweetener if desired)

- approx. 289 calories

OPTIONAL MIDMORNING SNACK

10–20 almonds or walnuts
8 ounces water or non-caloric beverage

LUNCH

Hearty Bean Soup (page 107)
1 slice whole grain bread with extra-virgin olive oil or 1 teaspoon vegetable
  spread (trans fat–free canola/olive oil spread)
3 fresh apricots
8 ounces water or non-caloric beverage

- approx. 414 calories

OPTIONAL MIDDAY SNACK

1 apple
8 ounces water or non-caloric beverage

DINNER

4 tablespoons hummus
½ (6-inch) whole wheat pita loaf, split open, sprayed with extra-virgin olive oil and herb seasonings of choice, and toasted until crispy in the oven or microwave
4 tomato wedges topped with slivers of red onion, freshly grated mozzarella cheese, chopped fresh cilantro, and drizzled with aged balsamic vinegar and 1 teaspoon extra-virgin olive oil.
Fettuccine with Smoked Salmon and Basil Pesto (page 212)
Peach Marsala Compote (page 296)
1 or 2 (4-ounce) glasses of red wine or purple grape juice
8 ounces water
Coffee or tea (soy or non-fat milk, trans fat–free coffee creamer, and non-caloric sweetener if desired)

- APPROX. 774 CALORIES

OPTIONAL EVENING SNACK

2 Meringue Cookies (page 316)
Green tea or 8 ounces water

DAY 6

BREAKFAST

4 ounces vegetable or fruit juice
½ cup dry oatmeal, cooked and sweetened with non-caloric sweetener if desired
1 tablespoon seedless black raisins
1 medium orange, sliced
8 ounces water
Coffee or tea (soy or non-fat milk, trans fat–free coffee creamer, and non-caloric sweetener if desired)

- APPROX. 292 CALORIES

OPTIONAL MIDMORNING SNACK

10–20 almonds or walnuts
8 ounces water or non-caloric beverage

LUNCH

Veggie Wrap (page 271)
Roasted Peppers (page 237)
6–8 marinated mixed olives
1 medium fresh pear, peach, or apple
8 ounces water or non-caloric beverage

• APPROX. 601 CALORIES

OPTIONAL MIDDAY SNACK

1 apple
8 ounces water or non-caloric beverage

DINNER

1 jumbo clove Roasted Garlic (page 335)
½ (6-inch) whole wheat pita loaf, split open, sprayed with olive oil and herb
*   seasonings, and toasted until crispy in the oven or microwave*
Mediterranean Mixed Greens (page 79)
Baked Tilapia (page 176)
Classic Spinach and Pine Nuts (page 238)
Strawberries Amaretto (page 308)
8 ounces water
1 or 2 (4-ounce) glasses of red wine or purple grape juice coffee or tea (soy or
*   non-fat milk, trans fat–free coffee creamer, and non-caloric sweetener if*
*   desired)*

• APPROX. 597 CALORIES

OPTIONAL EVENING SNACK

2 Meringue Cookies (page 316)
Green tea or 8 ounces water

DAY 7

BREAKFAST

4 ounces vegetable or fruit juice

½ cup egg whites with diced red onion, tomato, and green bell peppers cooked into an omelet

1 slice whole wheat toast with extra-virgin olive oil or 1 teaspoon vegetable spread (trans fat–free canola/olive oil spread)

1 teaspoon fruit jam

1 purple plum

8 ounces water

Coffee or tea (soy or non-fat milk, trans fat–free coffee creamer, and non-caloric sweetener if desired)

• APPROX. 230 CALORIES

OPTIONAL MIDMORNING SNACK

10–20 almonds or walnuts

8 ounces water or non-caloric beverage

LUNCH

Eggplant Soup (page 112)

1 slice whole grain crusty bread, drizzled with extra-virgin olive oil and herb seasonings of choice

1 large kiwi fruit, sliced

½ cup fresh strawberries, sliced

8 ounces water or non-caloric beverage

• APPROX. 420 CALORIES

OPTIONAL MIDDAY SNACK

1 apple

8 ounces water or non-caloric beverage

DINNER

1 slice whole grain bread with extra-virgin olive oil and herb seasonings of choice

6–8 marinated assorted olives

Broccoli with Fresh Garlic (page 243)

Fettuccine with Sundried Tomatoes and Goat Cheese (page 185)
Fresh Fruit Kabobs and Cinnamon Honey Dip (page 299)
8 ounces water
1 or 2 (4-ounce) glasses of red wine or purple grape juice
Coffee or tea (soy or non-fat milk, trans fat–free coffee creamer, and non-
*   caloric sweetener if desired)*

* APPROX. 1050 CALORIES

OPTIONAL EVENING SNACK

1 apple or orange
8 ounces water

DAY 8

BREAKFAST

4 ounces vegetable or fruit juice
½ cup dry oatmeal, cooked and sweetened with non-caloric sweetener if desired
1 tablespoon seedless dark raisins
1 small banana, sliced
8 ounces water
Coffee or tea (soy or non-fat milk, trans fat–free coffee creamer, and non-
*   caloric sweetener if desired)*

* APPROX. 323 CALORIES

OPTIONAL MIDMORNING SNACK

10–20 almonds or walnuts
8 ounces water or non-caloric beverage

LUNCH

Easy Couscous Parsley Salad (page 91)
½ (6-inch) whole wheat pita loaf, split open, sprayed with olive oil and herb
*   seasonings, and toasted until crispy in the oven or microwave*
Fresh fruit in plain low-fat yogurt
8 ounces water or non-caloric beverage

* APPROX. 331 CALORIES

OPTIONAL MIDDAY SNACK

1 apple

8 ounces water or non-caloric beverage

DINNER

4 large pre-cooked shrimp with tails

2 tablespoons cocktail sauce

Avocado Salad (page 93)

½ (6-inch) whole wheat pita loaf, split open, sprayed with olive oil and herb seasonings of choice, and toasted until crispy in the oven or microwave

1 tablespoon mustard if desired

1 tablespoon catsup, if desired

1 slice raw onion

1 slice tomato

Mom's Turkey Burger (page 211)

½-inch slice honeydew or cantaloupe

8 ounces water

1 or 2 (4-ounce) glasses of red wine or purple grape juice

Coffee or tea (soy or non-fat milk, trans fat–free coffee creamer, and non-caloric sweetener if desired)

- APPROX. 714 CALORIES

OPTIONAL EVENING SNACK

1 apple or orange

8 ounces water

DAY 9

BREAKFAST

4 ounces vegetable or fruit juice

2 slices whole wheat toast

2 tablespoons fresh chunky peanut butter

2 teaspoons honey

½ ruby red grapefruit, sweetened with non-caloric sweetener

8 ounces water

Coffee or tea (soy or non-fat milk, trans fat–free coffee creamer, and non-

caloric sweetener if desired)

• APPROX. 385 CALORIES

OPTIONAL MIDMORNING SNACK

10–20 almonds or walnuts
8 ounces water or non-caloric beverage

LUNCH

Chicken Escarole Soup (page 110)
1 slice whole grain crusty bread
⅛ wedge honeydew
8 ounces water or non-caloric beverage

• APPROX. 259 CALORIES

OPTIONAL MIDDAY SNACK

1 apple
8 ounces water or a non-caloric beverage

DINNER

2 Stuffed Grape Leaves (Dolmas) with lemon slices (page 336)
½ (6-inch) whole wheat pita loaf, split open, sprayed with olive oil and herb
* seasonings of choice, and toasted until crispy in the oven or microwave*
6–8 marinated assorted olives
Baked Eggplant with Garlic and Basil (page 257)
Steamed Sea Bass (page 169)
Cantaloupe Sorbet (page 303)
8 ounces water
1 or 2 (4-ounce) glasses of red wine or purple grape juice
Coffee or tea (soy or non-fat milk, trans fat–free coffee creamer, and non-
* caloric sweetener if desired)*

• APPROX. 662 CALORIES

OPTIONAL EVENING SNACK

2 Meringue Cookies (page 316)
Green tea or 8 ounces water

DAY 10

BREAKFAST

4 ounces vegetable or fruit juice
1 slice whole wheat toast with extra-virgin olive oil or 1 teaspoon vegetable spread (trans fat–free canola/olive oil spread)
1 teaspoon fruit jam
½ cup plain low-fat yogurt, sweetened with non-caloric sweetener
½ cup fresh blueberries or strawberries
8 ounces water
Coffee or tea (soy or non-fat milk, trans fat–free coffee creamer, and non-caloric sweetener if desired)

- APPROX. 289 CALORIES

OPTIONAL MIDMORNING SNACK

10–20 almonds or walnuts
8 ounces water or non-caloric beverage

LUNCH

Chilled Stuffed Pasta Shells (page 239)
10–20 seedless grapes
1 large fresh tangerine
8 ounces water or non-caloric beverage

- APPROX. 292 CALORIES

OPTIONAL MIDDAY SNACK

1 apple
8 ounces water or non-caloric beverage

DINNER

1 jumbo clove Roasted Garlic (page 335)
½ (6-inch) whole wheat pita loaf, split open, sprayed with extra-virgin olive oil and herb seasonings of choice, and toasted until crispy in the oven or microwave

Roasted Peppers (page 237)
Spicy Shrimp with Angel Hair Pasta (page 164)
Crème de Banana Baked Apples (page 302)
8 ounces water
1 or 2 (4-ounce) glasses of red wine or purple grape juice
Coffee or tea (soy or non-fat milk, trans fat–free coffee creamer, and non-caloric sweetener if desired)

- APPROX. 735 CALORIES

OPTIONAL EVENING SNACK

1 apple or orange
8 ounces water

DAY 11

BREAKFAST

4 ounces vegetable or fruit juice
½ cup dry oatmeal, cooked and sweetened with non-caloric sweetener if desired
1 tablespoon seedless dark raisins
1 medium orange, sliced
8 ounces water
Coffee or tea (soy or non-fat milk, trans fat–free coffee creamer, and non-caloric sweetener if desired)

- APPROX. 292 CALORIES

OPTIONAL MIDMORNING SNACK

10–20 almonds or walnuts
8 ounces water or non-caloric beverage

LUNCH

Garlicky Cannellini Beans (page 259)
½ (6-inch) whole wheat pita loaf, split open, sprayed with extra-virgin olive oil and herb seasonings of choice, and toasted in the oven or microwave
1 medium apple sliced and drizzled with 1 teaspoon honey

8 ounces water or non-caloric beverage

- APPROX. 389 CALORIES

OPTIONAL MIDDAY SNACK

10–20 almonds or walnuts
8 ounces water or non-caloric beverage

DINNER

Light Caesar Salad (page 85)
1 slice whole grain bread or whole grain dinner roll
1 tablespoon extra-virgin olive oil and a splash of aged balsamic vinegar for
dipping, seasoned with freshly ground pepper if desired
Lemon Garlic Asparagus (page 246)
Meatless Lasagna (page 209)
Strawberry and Poached Pears (page 292)
8 ounces water
1 or 2 (4-ounce) glasses of red wine or purple grape juice
Coffee or tea (soy or non-fat milk, trans fat–free coffee creamer, and non-
caloric sweetener if desired)

- APPROX. 790 CALORIES

OPTIONAL EVENING SNACK

2 Meringue Cookies (page 316)
Green tea or 8 ounces water

DAY 12

BREAKFAST

4 ounces vegetable or fruit juice
½ cup egg whites with diced onions, tomato, and green bell peppers cooked
into an omelet
1 slice whole wheat toast with extra-virgin olive oil or 1 teaspoon vegetable
spread (trans fat–free canola/olive oil spread)
1 teaspoon fruit jam
½ small banana

8 ounces water
Coffee or tea (soy or non-fat milk, trans fat–free coffee creamer, and non-caloric sweetener if desired)

- APPROX. 230 CALORIES

OPTIONAL MIDMORNING SNACK

10–20 almonds or walnuts
8 ounces water or non-caloric beverage

LUNCH

Smoked Fish and Roasted Pepper Sandwich (page 279)
½ cup fresh raspberries
½ cup plain low-fat yogurt, non-caloric sweetener if desired
8 ounces water or non-caloric beverage

- APPROX. 322 CALORIES

OPTIONAL MIDDAY SNACK

1 apple
8 ounces water or non-caloric beverage

DINNER

Mediterranean Mixed Greens (page 79)
Tomato and Fresh Parmesan Cheese Bruschetta (page 338)
1 slice crusty toasted French bread with extra-virgin olive oil
Fresh vegetable of choice (flavor with olive oil or trans fat–free canola/olive oil as desired)
Bow Tie Pasta with Eggplant and Black Olives (page 181)
Sweet Italian Rice Pudding (page 301)
8 ounces water
1 or 2 (4-ounce) glasses of red wine or purple grape juice
Coffee or tea (soy or non-fat milk, trans fat–free coffee creamer, and non-caloric sweetener if desired)

- APPROX. 984 CALORIES

OPTIONAL EVENING SNACK

1 apple or orange
8 ounces water

DAY 13

BREAKFAST

4 ounces vegetable or fruit juice
2 slices whole wheat toast
2 tablespoons fresh chunky peanut butter
2 teaspoons honey
½ ruby red grapefruit, sweetened with non-caloric sweetener if desired
8 ounces water
Coffee or tea (soy or non-fat milk, trans fat–free coffee creamer, and non-caloric sweetener if desired)

- APPROX. 385 CALORIES

OPTIONAL MIDMORNING SNACK

10–20 almonds or walnuts
8 ounces water or non-caloric beverage

LUNCH

Chickpeas and Garden Vegetables (page 77)
½ (6-inch) whole wheat pita loaf, split open, sprayed with olive oil and herb seasonings of choice, and toasted in the oven or microwave
1 medium orange, sliced
8 ounces water or non-caloric beverage

- APPROX. 325 CALORIES

OPTIONAL MIDDAY SNACK

1 apple
8 ounces water or non-caloric beverage

DINNER

1 jumbo clove Roasted Garlic (page 335)
½ (6-inch) whole wheat pita loaf, split open, sprayed with olive oil and herb seasonings of choice, and toasted until crispy in the oven or microwave
6–8 marinated assorted olives
Steamed Artichoke (page 262)
Trout Almandine (page 215)
Strawberries and Balsamic Syrup (page 305)
8 ounces water
1 or 2 (4-ounce) glasses of red wine or purple grape juice
Coffee or tea (soy or non-fat milk, trans fat–free coffee creamer, and non-caloric sweetener if desired)

* APPROX. 578 CALORIES

OPTIONAL EVENING SNACK

2 Meringue Cookies (page 316)
Green tea or 8 ounces water

DAY 14

BREAKFAST

4 ounces vegetable or fruit juice
½ cup dry oatmeal, cooked and sweetened with non-caloric sweetener if desired
1 tablespoon seedless dark raisins
1 medium orange, sliced
8 ounces water
Coffee or tea (soy or non-fat milk, trans fat–free coffee creamer, and non-caloric sweetener if desired)

* APPROX. 292 CALORIES

OPTIONAL MIDMORNING SNACK

10–20 almonds or walnuts
8 ounces water or non-caloric beverage

LUNCH

Spicy Mushroom Wrap (page 277)
1 medium fresh peach
8 ounces water or non-caloric beverage

- APPROX. 544 CALORIES

OPTIONAL MIDDAY SNACK

1 apple
8 ounces water or non-caloric beverage

DINNER

1 jumbo clove Roasted Garlic (page 335)
½ (6-inch) whole wheat pita loaf, split open, sprayed with olive oil and herb
seasonings of choice, and toasted until crispy in the oven or microwave
Goat Cheese Stuffed Tomato (page 74)
Fresh vegetable of choice (flavor with olive oil or vegetable spread as desired)
Pasta with Red Clam Sauce (page 182)
Drunken Peaches (page 306)
8 ounces water
1 or 2 (4-ounce) glasses of red wine or purple grape juice
Coffee or tea (soy or non-fat milk, trans fat–free coffee creamer, and non-
caloric sweetener if desired)

- APPROX. 830 CALORIES

OPTIONAL EVENING SNACK

2 Meringue Cookies (page 316)
Green tea or 8 ounces water

A Guide to
Cooking Method Terminology

Boiling......................... cooking in water or other liquid at 212 degrees

Simmering .... cooking in water or other liquid at a temperature less than boiling point (around 180–210 degrees)

Steaming...................... cooking by steam that is generated by a small amount of water or other liquid

Stewing....................... simmering in just enough liquid to cover food (usually used to cook tender cuts of beef)

Broiling....................... cooking in an oven, either over or under direct heat, with the oven door slightly ajar

Pan broiling .... cooking in a ridged heavy skillet oiled only enough to keep the food from sticking

Baking or *Roasting* ...... these are the same thing, cooking in a closed-door oven

Sautéing....................... rapid cooking in a pan on a stovetop using very little oil

Frying.......................... cooking in a pan on a stovetop where the food is bathed in oil

Fricasseeing .... a combination of sautéing and stewing or steaming

Salads

GREEK OLIVE AND FETA CHEESE PASTA
(MAKES 4 SERVINGS)

4½ ounces ziti pasta
3 ounces crumbled feta cheese
10 small Greek olives, pitted and coarsely chopped
¼ cup fresh, coarsely chopped basil leaves
2 cloves garlic, finely minced
1 tablespoon extra-virgin olive oil
¼ teaspoon finely chopped hot pepper
½ red bell pepper, diced
½ yellow bell pepper, diced
2 plum tomatoes, seeded and diced

Bring water to a boil, add pasta, and cook pasta until *al dente*. Remove from heat, drain pasta, and return to pot, drizzling with scant amount of olive oil to keep pasta from sticking together. Set aside. In a large serving bowl combine feta cheese, olives, basil, garlic, olive oil, and hot peppers, then set aside for 30 minutes. Add cooked pasta, red and yellow bell peppers, and tomato; toss ingredients well. Cover and refrigerate for at least 1 hour, until well chilled. Toss again before serving.

This salad goes well as a side dish to grilled lamb or fish.

Approx. 235 calories per serving
7g protein, 10g total fat, 1g saturated fat, 0 trans fat,
27g carbohydrates, 18mg cholesterol, 98mg sodium, 2g fiber

GOAT CHEESE STUFFED TOMATOES
(MAKES 2 SERVINGS)

6–8 leaves arugula
2 medium ripe tomatoes
3 ounces crumbled feta cheese
Salt and freshly ground pepper to taste
Balsamic vinegar
Extra-virgin olive oil
1 red onion, very thinly sliced
Fresh chopped parsley

Place 3–4 leaves arugula in the center of each salad plate. Cut tops (about ¼ inch) off the tomatoes. With a paring knife, core out the center of the tomatoes, about ½ inch deep. Fill tomatoes with crumbled feta cheese, add salt and pepper to taste, and drizzle with balsamic vinegar and extra-virgin olive oil. Garnish with red onion slices and chopped parsley. Serve at room temperature.

Approx. 142 calories per serving
7g protein, 13g total fat, 3g saturated fat, 0 trans fat,
7g carbohydrates, 37mg cholesterol, 485mg sodium, 1g fiber

CLASSIC TABBOULEH
(MAKES 4–6 SERVINGS AS DINNER SALAD OR 8–10 AS APPETIZER)

¾ cup bulgur
1½ cups water
2 cups freshly chopped parsley
¾ cup chopped scallions, white and green parts
½ red bell pepper, diced
½ green bell pepper, diced
½ cup finely chopped fresh mint
½ cup fresh lemon juice
½ cup extra-virgin olive oil
Sea salt and freshly ground pepper to taste
3 ripe plum tomatoes, peeled, seeded, and diced
1 large cucumber, peeled, seeded, and diced

In a small saucepan soak bulgur in water for 30 minutes. Drain bulgur through a sieve and allow it to dry thoroughly. Clean parsley under cold running water and press gently between paper towels to dry. Place bulgur, parsley, scallions, peppers, and mint in a large bowl. Stir to mix well. In a separate bowl whisk together lemon juice and oil. Season bulgur mixture with salt and pepper. Add lemon mixture to bulgur—only enough to make salad moist (not runny)—and toss. Fold in tomatoes and cucumbers, then cover and chill. Serve on a bed of greens, with seasoned pita wedges for dipping.

This salad goes well with toasted, herb-seasoned whole wheat pita triangles.

Approx. 177 calories per serving
3g protein, 21g total fat, 2g saturated fat, 0 trans fat,
19g carbohydrates, 0 cholesterol, 23mg sodium, 4g fiber

SAVORY GREEK WHITE FAVA BEAN SALAD
(MAKES 4 SERVINGS)

1¼ cups dried white fava beans
2–3 fresh sage leaves
Salt to taste
2 cloves garlic, finely minced
1 small onion, finely chopped
1 celery stalk, finely chopped
3 tablespoons fresh lemon juice
½ teaspoon dried oregano
3 tablespoons extra-virgin olive oil
4½ tablespoons red wine vinegar
Freshly ground pepper to taste

Soak the beans overnight in fresh water (water must cover the beans by twice its volume). In the morning, drain beans, rinse with fresh water, and drain a second time. Combine drained beans and 1 quart of fresh water in a large pot; bring to a boil. Add sage, cover pot, and cook for about 45 minutes. Gently stir and add salt to taste. Continue cooking for about another 15 minutes, until beans are soft but not mushy. Remove from heat and drain. Let beans cool slightly, then toss with garlic, onions, celery, lemon juice, oregano, oil, and vinegar. Add freshly ground pepper to taste, and chill for one hour or more before serving.

Approx. 253 calories per serving
12g protein, 11g total fat, 1g saturated fat, 0 trans fat,
28g carbohydrates, 0 cholesterol, 15mg sodium, 12g fiber

CHICKPEAS AND GARDEN VEGETABLES
(MAKES 4 SERVINGS)

2 tablespoons freshly squeezed lemon juice
2 cloves garlic, finely minced
1 tablespoon fresh basil leaf, snipped
⅛ teaspoon freshly ground pepper
1 (15-ounce) can chickpeas, rinsed and well drained
2 cups coarsely chopped fresh broccoli
½ cup sliced fresh carrots
1 (7½-ounce) can diced tomatoes (do not drain)
1 cup cubed part-skim mozzarella cheese

In a large serving bowl combine lemon juice, garlic, basil, and ground pepper. Stir in beans, broccoli, carrots, tomatoes with juice, and cheese. Toss ingredients, mixing well. Cover and refrigerate for at least 4 hours.

Approx. 195 calories per serving
16g protein, 7g total fat, 2g saturated fat, 0 trans fat,
24g carbohydrates, 17mg cholesterol, 411mg sodium, 2g fiber

TANGY ORANGE ROASTED ASPARAGUS SALAD
(MAKES 6 SERVINGS)

1 pound fresh asparagus, trimmed and cut into ½-inch diagonal pieces
4 tablespoons extra-virgin olive oil
Salt to taste
4 tablespoons fresh, sweet, no-pulp orange juice
1 tablespoon freshly squeezed lime juice
2 cloves finely minced garlic
Freshly ground pepper to taste
7 cups chopped fresh romaine lettuce
3 tablespoons toasted pine nuts
1 tablespoon minced fresh basil leaf
Freshly grated Romano cheese (optional)

Toss asparagus with 2 tablespoons of olive oil and salt to taste. Arrange asparagus in a baking dish in a single layer and place in oven. Roast until tender crispy, about 10 minutes. Set aside. In a bowl, briskly whisk orange juice, lime juice, garlic, and remaining 2 tablespoons of olive oil; salt and pepper to taste. When ready to serve, divide lettuce into 6 servings, arrange on salad plates, and top with asparagus. Briefly whisk the dressing and pour over lettuce and asparagus salad. Top with toasted pine nuts and fresh minced basil. Garnish with a small amount of grated cheese if desired.

To toast pine nuts in the oven:

Place the nuts in one layer on a nonstick baking sheet. Bake at 375 degrees, stirring occasionally, until lightly browned. Remove from oven and allow to cool.

Approx. 124 calories per serving
4g protein, 10g total fat, 2g saturated fat, 0 trans fat,
6g carbohydrates, 0 cholesterol, 16mg sodium, 3g fiber

MEDITERRANEAN MIXED GREENS
(MAKES 4–6 SERVINGS)

6 cups assorted fresh mixed greens (such as arugula, radicchio, baby spinach,
*   watercress, and romaine)*
1 small red onion, thinly sliced and separated into rings
20 firm cherry tomatoes, halved
¼ cup chopped walnuts
¼ cup dried cranberries

For Dressing:

2 tablespoons balsamic vinegar
4 tablespoons extra-virgin olive oil
1 tablespoon water
½ teaspoon crushed dried oregano
2 cloves garlic, finely minced
Crumbled feta cheese (optional)
Freshly ground pepper to taste

In a large salad bowl, combine greens, onion, tomatoes, walnuts, and cranberries. Gently toss.

Dressing:

Combine vinegar, oil, water, oregano, and garlic; shake well. Pour dressing over salad and toss lightly to coat. Garnish with feta cheese, if desired, and fresh pepper.

Approx. 140 calories per serving
2g protein, 12g total fat, 1g saturated fat, 0 trans fat,
6g carbohydrates, 0 cholesterol, 47mg sodium, 1g fiber

NORTH AFRICAN ZUCCHINI SALAD
(MAKES 4 SERVINGS)

1 pound firm green zucchini, thinly sliced
Juice from 1 large lemon
2 cloves garlic, finely minced
½ teaspoon ground cumin
1 tablespoon extra-virgin olive oil
1½ tablespoons plain low-fat yogurt
Salt and freshly ground pepper to taste
Finely chopped parsley
Crumbled feta cheese (optional)

Steam zucchini until crispy tender, roughly 2–5 minutes. Rinse under cold water and drain well. In a large salad bowl, mix the lemon juice, garlic, cumin, oil, yogurt, and salt and pepper to taste. Add zucchini and gently toss. Chill in the refrigerator for 45 minutes to 1 hour before serving. Garnish with parsley and cheese if desired.

Approx. 66 calories per serving
4g protein, 4g total fat, <0.5g saturated fat, 0 trans fat,
6g carbohydrates, 0 cholesterol, 22mg sodium, 1g fiber

GREENS WITH CHEESE MEDALLIONS
(MAKES 6 SERVINGS)

6 ounces soft goat cheese, log style
½ cup extra-virgin olive oil, divided in half
¼ cup plain bread crumbs
2 tablespoons freshly crushed garlic
Olive oil cooking spray
6 cups (roughly 16–18 ounces) mixed greens such as escarole, red and green
*   leaf lettuce, radicchio, and endive, washed and well dried*
1 cup halved cherry tomatoes
2 tablespoons red wine vinegar
2 teaspoons Dijon mustard
Salt and freshly ground pepper to taste
Finely chopped pecans (optional)

Preheat broiler. Cut goat cheese log into 6 equal pieces and place cheese medallions in a bowl containing ¼ cup olive oil; lightly swish mixture. Transfer the oil-laden cheese medallions to a bowl containing a mixture of bread crumbs and crushed garlic. Coat medallions on both sides with bread crumbs and garlic mixture. Lightly spray a baking sheet with olive oil spray and place medallions on sheet; broil until golden brown and crisp, 1–2 minutes per side. Toss greens with tomatoes, divide into 6 portions, and top each portion with a cheese medallion. Combine the remaining ¼ cup olive oil, red wine vinegar, and Dijon mustard in a bottle and shake to mix well. Drizzle mixture over salads. Add salt and pepper to taste. Garnish with pecans, if desired, before serving.

Approx. 204 calories per serving
6g protein, 25g total fat, 6.9g saturated fat, 0 trans fat,
6g carbohydrates, 0 cholesterol, 159mg sodium, 1g fiber

FENNEL SALAD
(MAKES 4–6 SERVINGS)

1 large clove garlic, halved
1 large fennel bulb, thinly sliced
½ English cucumber, thinly sliced
1 tablespoon minced fresh chives
8 large radishes, thinly sliced
3 tablespoons extra-virgin olive oil
2½ tablespoons freshly squeezed lemon juice
Salt and freshly ground pepper to taste
Marinated mixed olives (optional)

Rub the inside of a large bowl with garlic. Add fennel, cucumber, chives, and radishes. In a separate bowl whisk together olive oil, fresh lemon juice, and salt and pepper to taste. Pour olive oil mixture over salad and toss to mix. Garnish with marinated olives if desired.

Approx. 76 calories per serving
0 protein, 10g total fat, 1g saturated fat, 0 trans fat,
3g carbohydrates, 2mg cholesterol, 20mg sodium, 1g fiber

TUNISIAN CARROT SALAD
(MAKES 6 SERVINGS)

10 medium carrots, peeled and sliced into ½-inch-thick slices
5 teaspoons freshly minced garlic
Salt to taste
2 teaspoons caraway seed
1 tablespoon Harissa (page 352)
6 tablespoons cider vinegar
¼ cup extra-virgin olive oil
1 cup crumbled feta cheese
20 pitted Kalamata olives

In a medium saucepan filled with water, cook carrots until tender. Drain and cool under cold running water, then drain again and place in a bowl. Combine garlic, salt, and caraway seed in a mortar and grind until it forms a rough paste, then pulse the paste in a food processor. Add Harissa and vinegar and mix well. Mash the carrots. Add the garlic-caraway mixture to Harissa, blend well, and mix in olive oil. Add ¾ of the cheese and olives and toss again. Place salad in a shallow bowl and garnish with remaining feta cheese and olives.

Approx. 138 calories per serving
7g protein, 15g total fat, 5g saturated fat, 0 trans fat,
13g carbohydrates, 0 cholesterol, 643mg sodium, 17g fiber

CLASSIC GREEK SALAD
(MAKES 6 SERVINGS)

¼ cup extra-virgin olive oil
3 tablespoons red wine vinegar
2 cloves garlic, finely minced
1 tablespoon dried oregano
Pinch of low-calorie baking sweetener
Salt and fresh black pepper to taste
½ head of escarole, shredded
6 large firm tomatoes, quartered
½ English cucumber, peeled, seeded, and thinly sliced
1 medium red bell pepper, seeded and sliced
½ red onion, sliced
½ pound Greek feta cheese, cut into small cubes
20 Greek black olives
¼ cup freshly chopped Italian parsley

Whisk together oil, vinegar, garlic, oregano, sweetener, salt, and black pepper, and set aside. Combine escarole, tomatoes, cucumbers, pepper, onion, and cheese in a large salad bowl and toss. Drizzle oil mixture over salad and toss again. Scatter olives and parsley over salad and serve.

Approx. 268 calories per serving
23g protein, 17g total fat, 7g saturated fat, 0 trans fat,
44g carbohydrates, 0 cholesterol, 595mg sodium, 3g fiber

LIGHT CAESAR SALAD
(MAKES 6 SERVINGS)

1–2 bunches packaged pre-cleaned romaine lettuce, torn in pieces
½ cup non-fat plain yogurt
2 teaspoons lemon juice
2½ teaspoons balsamic vinegar
1 teaspoon Worcestershire sauce
2 cloves freshly minced garlic
½ teaspoon anchovy paste
½ cup grated Parmesan cheese
10 small pitted black olives, chopped

Clean and pat dry romaine lettuce and place in large salad bowl. In a blender mix yogurt, lemon juice, vinegar, Worcestershire sauce, garlic, anchovy paste, and ¼ cup Parmesan cheese until smooth. Pour mixture over lettuce and toss. Garnish with remaining cheese and olives.

Approx. 49 calories per serving
4g protein, 1g total fat, <0.1g saturated fat, 0 trans fat,
4g carbohydrates, 4mg cholesterol, 112mg sodium, 1g fiber

MOROCCAN EGGPLANT SALAD
(MAKES 4–6 SERVINGS)

1 large unpeeled eggplant (about 1 pound), cubed
3 cloves garlic, finely chopped
5 cups water
1 teaspoon salt
3 tablespoons extra-virgin olive oil
2 large tomatoes, chopped
1 teaspoon cumin
1 teaspoon paprika
¼ cup lemon juice

In a pot, place the eggplant cubes, roughly ⅓ of the garlic, water, and salt. Cover and boil for about 5–10 minutes, or until the eggplant is cooked but still firm. Drain cubes in a strainer and allow to cool. In a large skillet, heat 2 tablespoons olive oil. Add tomatoes, remaining garlic, cumin, and paprika. Stir while mashing with a fork until mixture is somewhat smooth. Remove from heat. Combine eggplant cubes with tomato mixture in a bowl; allow to slightly cool before covering. Refrigerate and chill for about 2 hours. Before serving, add lemon juice and remainder of olive oil, and toss gently.

Approx. 128 calories per serving
1g protein, 7g total fat, 1g saturated fat, 0 trans fat,
13g carbohydrates, 0 cholesterol, 561mg sodium, 4g fiber

SYRIAN CUCUMBER AND YOGURT SALAD
(MAKES 4 SERVINGS)

1½ teaspoons freshly crushed garlic
⅛ teaspoon minced fresh dill
Salt to taste
1 quart plain low-fat yogurt
2 English cucumbers, peeled and diced
2 tablespoons dried mint

In a bowl combine garlic, dill, and salt. Add yogurt and mix well. Stir in cucumbers and mint. Cover, and refrigerate until well chilled before serving.

Approx. 167 calories per serving
13g protein, 4g total fat, <0.5g saturated fat, 0 trans fat,
21g carbohydrates, 10mg cholesterol, 183mg sodium, 1g fiber

TUNISIAN TUNA SALAD
(MAKES 4 SERVINGS)

3 large ripe tomatoes, peeled
2 medium green bell peppers, seeded and sliced into thin rings
1 large cucumber, sliced
1 sweet onion, thinly sliced and separated into rings
2 hard-boiled eggs, shelled and divided into quarters
2 tablespoons fresh lemon juice
2 cloves garlic, minced
2 tablespoons red wine vinegar
1 tablespoon water
1 teaspoon Dijon mustard
2 tablespoons chopped fresh basil
¼ cup extra-virgin olive oil
1 (12-ounce) can water-packed white albacore tuna, drained and divided
  into 4 equal parts
Salt and freshly ground black pepper to taste
Capers, rinsed and drained, for garnish
Kalamata olives, chopped, for garnish

Divide tomatoes, peppers, cucumbers, onion rings, and eggs into 4 portions. On 4 individual salad platters first layer tomatoes, then cover with layers of pepper rings, cucumbers, and onions. Arrange eggs around edges of platters. In a small bowl, whisk the lemon juice, garlic, vinegar, water, mustard, and basil together until smooth. Gradually whisk in olive oil. Pour dressing over each salad platter. Place a scoop of tuna on the center of each salad, and add salt and ground pepper to taste. Garnish with capers and olives.

Approx. 306 calories per serving
27g protein, 17g total fat, 3g saturated fat, 0 trans fat,
13g carbohydrates, 132mg cholesterol, 332mg sodium, 3g fiber

FRESHLY CHOPPED SALAD WITH WALNUT DRESSING
(MAKES 6 SERVINGS)

3 medium ripe tomatoes, seeded and chopped
1 medium cucumber, peeled, seeded, and diced
1 large green bell pepper, seeded and diced
5 scallions, finely chopped
1 head iceberg lettuce
¼ cup fresh spearmint leaves, finely chopped
20 pitted Kalamata black olives

For Walnut Dressing:

2 slices Italian bread, soaked in water, squeezed dry, and crumbled
¼ cup finely minced shelled walnuts
½ teaspoon finely crushed garlic
¼ cup extra-virgin olive oil
Lemon juice, freshly squeezed, to taste
Salt to taste (optional)
Red hot pepper sauce to taste (optional)

In a large mixing bowl combine tomatoes, cucumber, green pepper, and chopped scallions. Add Walnut Dressing and toss thoroughly. Add salt to taste. Line a serving platter with lettuce leaves. Spoon salad mixture over cleaned and separated lettuce leaves, sprinkle with mint, and garnish with olives. Serve immediately.

Walnut Dressing:

In a blender or food processor add bread, walnuts, and garlic and blend while slowly adding olive oil. Gradually add lemon juice and beat until mixture is smooth. Add salt and hot pepper sauce to taste.

Approx. 195 calories per serving of salad plus dressing
4g protein, 16g total fat, 1g saturated fat, 0 trans fat,
13g carbohydrates, 0 cholesterol, 227mg sodium, 3g fiber

SIMPLE SPANISH SALAD
(MAKES 6 SERVINGS)

1 bag (2 bunches) cleaned and trimmed romaine lettuce, torn into bite-sized
   pieces
3 medium ripe tomatoes cut into ¼-inch wedges
1 large sweet onion, thinly sliced
1 green bell pepper, seeded and thinly sliced
1 red bell pepper, seeded and thinly sliced
¼ cup chopped and pitted marinated green olives
¼ cup chopped and pitted black olives
¼ cup extra-virgin olive oil
3 tablespoons balsamic vinegar
Salt and freshly ground pepper to taste

Place a bed of romaine lettuce on 6 chilled salad plates. Arrange tomatoes, onions, peppers, and olives on top of the lettuce on each plate. Mix olive oil and vinegar together; drizzle over salad. Add salt and pepper if desired and serve.

Approx. 107 calories per serving
2g protein, 9g total fat, 1g saturated fat, 0 trans fat,
7g carbohydrates, 0 cholesterol, 145mg sodium, 3g fiber

EASY COUSCOUS PARSLEY SALAD
(MAKES 4 SERVINGS)

¼ cup dry couscous
¼ cup water
2 tablespoons fresh lemon juice
2 teaspoons extra-virgin olive oil
¼ cup finely chopped fresh flat parsley leaves
2 tablespoons finely chopped fresh mint leaves
2 teaspoons lemon zest
2 tablespoons pine nuts
Salt and freshly ground pepper to taste
1 medium ripe tomato, peeled, seeded, and diced
2 heads Belgian endive, leaves for scooping
Whole wheat pita rounds, cut into wedges and toasted until crispy (optional)

Combine couscous with water and lemon juice in a medium bowl, and let stand for 1 hour. After 1 hour, add olive oil, parsley, mint, lemon zest, pine nuts, and salt and pepper to taste. Mix well. Mold couscous mixture into a mound in the center of a serving platter and garnish with tomato. Surround with endive leaves or toasted pita wedges if desired. Serve at room temperature.

Approx. 120 calories per serving
5g protein, 2g total fat, <0.5g saturated fat, 0 trans fat,
18g carbohydrate, 0 cholesterol, 65mg sodium, 9g fiber

SARDINE SALAD
(MAKES 4–6 SERVINGS)

8 ounces spiral-shaped pasta
¼ cup extra-virgin olive oil
1 medium onion, thinly sliced
2 cloves fresh garlic, minced
½ small hot pepper, seeded and finely chopped
⅓ cup freshly squeezed orange juice
¼ cup golden raisins
¼ cup toasted sliced almonds
16 jumbo pitted green olives, chopped
7½ ounces (2 cans) sardines in olive oil
Salt and freshly ground pepper to taste
Splash of lemon juice
4 tablespoons finely chopped fresh parsley
Finely shredded Parmesan cheese (optional)

Bring water to a boil, add pasta, and cook pasta until tender. Remove from heat, drain pasta, and return to pot, drizzling with scant amount of olive oil to keep pasta from sticking together. Heat olive oil in a large skillet; add onions, garlic, and hot peppers, and sauté until golden brown. Add orange juice and raisins, and bring to a boil. Remove from heat but keep warm. Combine toasted almonds and olives with onion mixture; stir together. Add sardines but try not to break them into pieces. Pour sardine mixture over pasta. Add salt and pepper and a splash of lemon juice to taste. Garnish with parsley and a small amount of cheese if desired. Serve at room temperature.

Approx. 467 calories per serving
31g protein, 26g total fat, 2g saturated fat, 0 trans fat,
38g carbohydrates, 60mg cholesterol, 288mg sodium, 1g fiber

AVOCADO SALAD
(MAKES 3 SERVINGS)

1 large ripe avocado, pitted and peeled
1 cup halved cherry tomatoes
2 tablespoons chopped fresh parsley
1 small onion, finely chopped
½ small hot pepper, finely chopped (optional)
2 teaspoons fresh lime juice
Salt and freshly ground pepper to taste

Cut avocado into bite-sized chunks. Combine tomatoes, parsley, onion, hot pepper, and lime juice. Toss well; add salt and pepper to taste. Add avocado and toss gently. Divide into 3 equal portions and serve.

Approx. 130 calories per serving
2g protein, 10g total fat, 2g saturated fat, 0 trans fat,
10g carbohydrates, 0 cholesterol, 110mg sodium, 4g fiber

PASTA AND SHRIMP SALAD
(MAKES 6 SERVINGS)

½ pound whole wheat fettuccine
16 large (about 1 pound) pre-cooked shrimp
12 pitted black olives, halved
6 cherry tomatoes, halved
½ cup diced roasted red peppers
¼ cup chopped fresh parsley
¼ cup chopped fresh basil
4 scallions, trimmed and sliced
¼ pound feta cheese, crumbled
Salt and freshly ground pepper to taste
Extra-virgin olive oil for drizzling

Fill a large pot with water and heat to boiling, add pasta, and cook until *al dente*. When ready, drain pasta well and transfer to a large serving bowl. Add cooked shrimp, olives, tomatoes, peppers, parsley, basil, scallions, and cheese to pasta. Toss to mix. Add salt and pepper if desired and drizzle with olive oil to lightly moisten pasta; serve.

Approx. 411 calories per serving
32g protein, 6g total fat, 2g saturated fat, 0 trans fat,
57g carbohydrates, 150mg cholesterol, 206mg sodium, 3g fiber

TANGY TANGERINE CRESS SALAD
(MAKES 4 SERVINGS)

4 large sweet tangerines
Juice from 1 fresh lemon
¼ cup extra-virgin olive oil
Sea salt and freshly ground pepper to taste
2 large bunches watercress (washed, with tough stems removed)
10 cherry tomatoes, halved
16 pitted Kalamata olives

Peel tangerines and separate sections. Remove any pits and squeeze sections to get ¼ cup of juice. Set sections aside. In a large bowl, whisk together tangerine juice, lemon juice, oil, salt, and ground pepper to taste. Pat watercress dry with paper towels to remove any excess water. Add watercress, tomatoes, and olives to tangerine sections and toss with oil mixture. Serve immediately on chilled salad plates.

Approx. 195 calories per serving
3g protein, 16g total fat, 2g saturated fat, 0 trans fat,
14g carbohydrates, 0 cholesterol, 125mg sodium, 3g fiber

TOASTED CAPRI SALAD
(MAKES 4 SERVINGS)

1 large firm ripe tomato, cut into 8 thin slices
8 thin slices of red onion
1 (roughly 8-ounce) ball of fresh mozzarella cheese, cut into 8 slices
12 pitted Kalamata olives, halved
8 whole fresh basil leaves, garnish for plates
Aged balsamic vinegar to drizzle
Extra-virgin olive oil to drizzle
Sea salt and freshly ground pepper to taste
Freshly chopped basil for garnish

Preheat oven to broil. Divide first 4 ingredients into four equal portions. Alternate ingredients starting with tomato, onion, cheese, and top with a few olives to make 4 separate stacks. Place stacks in an oven-safe dish about 4 inches under broiler, and broil for about 2–3 minutes or until cheese partially melts. Remove from oven. Place 2 whole basil leaves on each plate and top with toasted salad stack. Drizzle small amount of vinegar and oil over each salad, add salt and pepper if desired, garnish with chopped basil, and serve.

Approx. 111 calories per serving
6g protein, 8g total fat, 4g saturated fat, 0 trans fat,
3g carbohydrates, 20mg cholesterol, 117mg sodium, <1g fiber

ENDIVE SPINACH SALAD
(MAKES 6 SERVINGS)

Olive oil cooking spray
½ cup chopped toasted walnuts
¼ cup extra-virgin olive oil
4 tablespoons freshly chopped shallots
2 tablespoons white wine vinegar
1 tablespoon pure maple syrup
Salt to taste
¼ teaspoon freshly ground pepper
1 (10-ounce) bag cleaned fresh spinach
2 heads Belgian endive
1½ tablespoons chopped dried cranberry
¼ cup crumbled Danish blue cheese

Spray a small heavy-bottomed skillet with cooking spray and lightly toast walnuts over medium heat. Stir constantly to keep from burning. Remove from heat and set aside. In a small bowl, whisk together oil, shallots, vinegar, syrup, salt, and pepper. Set aside to marry flavors. Place cleaned spinach in a large salad bowl. Cut endive on the diagonal into thin slices with a sharp knife and add to spinach. Add cranberries and walnuts to spinach and toss all ingredients with dressing. Sprinkle salad with cheese and serve.

Approx. 244 calories per serving
6g protein, 18g total fat, 3g saturated fat, 0 trans fat,
29g carbohydrates, 4mg cholesterol, 108mg sodium, 3g fiber

ARUGULA AND ASIAN PEAR SALAD
(MAKES 4 SERVINGS)

⅓ cup fresh grapefruit juice
⅓ cup fresh orange juice
3 tablespoons extra-virgin olive oil + enough to drizzle
1 small shallot, finely chopped
16 raw almonds, chopped
Dash of garlic powder
1 (6-ounce) bag arugula
1 ripe but firm Asian pear, halved and cored
¼ cup crumbled blue cheese
Salt and freshly ground pepper to taste

Whisk together both juices, olive oil, and shallots, and set aside to marry flavors. In a small skillet over medium heat, add chopped almonds, garlic powder, and a drizzle of olive oil. Toast almonds but do not burn; set aside. Divide arugula into four portions on salad plates. Slice pear into 16 slices and top each plate of arugula with 4 pear slices. Drizzle each salad with dressing, including bits of shallots. Scatter on blue cheese, toasted almonds, and salt and pepper to taste, and serve.

Approx. 208 calories per serving
5g protein, 16g total fat, 3g saturated fat, 0 trans fat,
10g carbohydrates, 6mg cholesterol, 101mg sodium, 3g fiber

Soups

EGG-LEMON PASTA SOUP
(MAKES 4 SERVINGS)

4 cups low-sodium, fat-free chicken broth
4 ounces ditalini pasta
½ cup egg substitute or 2 large whole eggs if desired
½ cup fresh lemon juice
Salt and freshly ground pepper to taste
4 tablespoons chopped fresh parsley
1 lemon, thinly sliced

In a medium saucepan, bring chicken broth to a boil. Add pasta; return to a boil, stirring once. Reduce to low, and simmer for 3–5 minutes. Remove from heat. Beat the eggs in a bowl, then beat in the lemon juice. Add a ladle of soup to this mixture and stir; transfer to soup pot. Heat soup on low heat, being careful not to curdle the eggs. Add salt and pepper to taste. Divide soup into 4 portions, garnish with parsley and lemon slices, and serve.

Approx. 161 calories per serving
10g protein, 2g total fat, <0.5g saturated fat, 0 trans fat,
65g carbohydrates, 5mg cholesterol, 197mg sodium, 1g fiber

BASIC LENTIL SOUP
(MAKES 6–8 SERVINGS)

4 cups low-sodium, fat-free chicken broth
4 cups water
1 cup split brown lentils, rinsed and drained
Salt and freshly ground pepper to taste
2 teaspoons ground cumin
¼ cup extra-virgin olive oil
2 medium yellow onions, finely chopped
4 large cloves garlic, finely chopped
2 ounces dry ditalini pasta
1 large firm ripe tomato, seeded and cut into chunks
10 ounces fresh escarole, washed and chopped (spinach)
1 cup finely chopped parsley
½ cup fresh lemon juice
Shredded Parmesan cheese for garnish (optional)

In a large pot add chicken broth and water, and bring to a boil. Add lentils, salt and pepper, and cumin, reduce heat to medium, and cook until lentils are tender. Do not overcook; beans should be tender but firm. While lentils are cooking, add oil to a skillet and sauté onions and garlic until golden brown. Stir mixture often to prevent burning; when browned, set aside. When lentils are almost tender, add pasta and cook until both are tender but not mushy. Reduce heat to a low simmer, and add garlic mixture, tomatoes, chopped escarole, parsley, and lemon juice. Simmer until escarole is cooked. Serve garnished with a small amount of cheese if desired.

Approx. 195 calories per serving
8g protein, 11g total fat, 1g saturated fat, 0 trans fat,
26g carbohydrates, 3mg cholesterol, 152mg sodium, 6g fiber

SAVORY MEDITERRANEAN CHICKPEA SOUP
(MAKES 6 SERVINGS)

2 cups water
4 cups low-sodium, fat-free chicken broth
4 cups canned chickpeas, rinsed with fresh water and drained
1 tablespoon extra-virgin olive oil
1 large onion, chopped
4–5 cloves fresh garlic minced
1 medium green bell pepper, chopped
1 teaspoon cayenne
2 teaspoons dried sage
2 teaspoons dried rosemary
1 teaspoon ground cinnamon
Salt and freshly ground pepper to taste
¼ cup crumbled low-fat feta cheese (optional)
2 tablespoons finely chopped fresh parsley

In a large pot combine water, broth, chickpeas, oil, onion, garlic, green pepper, cayenne, sage, rosemary, and cinnamon. Bring mixture to boil over medium heat, lower temperature, and simmer for 20 minutes, uncovered. Add salt and pepper to taste. Garnish with feta cheese and parsley.

Approx. 163 calories per serving
9g protein, 3g total fat, <0.5g saturated fat, 0 trans fat,
32g carbohydrates, 3mg cholesterol, 560mg sodium, 8g fiber

FRESH GARDEN GAZPACHO
(MAKES 4 SERVINGS)

4 cups chopped ripe peeled tomatoes
4 cloves garlic, chopped
½ red onion, chopped
1 green bell pepper, seeded and diced
¼ cup extra-virgin olive oil
2 tablespoons red wine vinegar
2 slices stale French sourdough bread
½ cup canned tomato juice
½ teaspoon cumin
½ small hot pepper, finely chopped
1 tablespoon chopped fresh basil
Salt and freshly ground pepper to taste
¼ cup green bell peppers and cucumbers for garnish, finely diced
Croutons (optional)
Plain low-fat sour cream or yogurt (optional)

In a food processor or blender, add tomatoes, garlic, onion, and green pepper. Blend until pureed. Add oil and vinegar, blend about 1 minute to mix. Soak bread in tomato juice, then add soaked bread mixture to blender. Add cumin, hot peppers, and basil. Blend for 2–3 minutes to mix well. Adjust with salt and pepper to taste. Chill for several hours. Serve very chilled, garnished with diced green peppers and cucumber. If desired, add croutons and a dollop of sour cream or yogurt.

Approx. 210 calories per serving
4g protein, 14g total fat, 2g saturated fat, 0 trans fat,
20g carbohydrates, 0 cholesterol, 201mg sodium, 3g fiber

CHILLY TOMATO SOUP
(MAKES 4 SERVINGS)

10 medium ripe tomatoes
½ tablespoon extra-virgin olive oil
4–5 cloves garlic, minced
2 tablespoons chopped onions
2 cups low-sodium, fat-free chicken broth
2 teaspoons low-calorie baking sweetener
½ teaspoon chopped fresh basil
Salt and freshly ground pepper to taste
8 scallions, chopped (optional)
2 cucumbers, diced (optional)
1 large green zucchini, diced (optional)

In a large pot of boiling water, dip tomatoes for 30 seconds, then immediately place tomatoes in cold water. Allow to sit until they can be handled. Skin tomatoes with a paring knife, cut in half crosswise, and remove seeds. Core and then cut into quarter pieces. In a blender or food processor, process tomatoes until pureed. In a skillet, heat olive oil and sauté garlic and onions until tender. Remove from heat. In a large bowl, combine pureed tomatoes, sautéed onion mixture, chicken broth, sweetener, basil, and salt and pepper, stirring to mix ingredients together. Refrigerate soup for 4–6 hours until well chilled. Garnish with scallions, cucumbers, and zucchini if desired.

Approx. 161 calories per serving
10g protein, <0.5g total fat, 0 saturated fat, 0 trans fat,
65g carbohydrates, 5mg cholesterol, 197mg sodium, 1g fiber

ITALIAN MINESTRONE SOUP WITH PESTO
(MAKES 6–8 SERVINGS)

1 cup dried cannellini beans

4 cups low-sodium, fat-free chicken broth

4 cups water

2 medium white potatoes, peeled and diced

2 ounces dry ditalini pasta

2 large carrots, chopped

3 stalks celery, chopped

½ cup chopped white onion

2 cloves garlic, minced

1 cup tomato juice

3 plum tomatoes, chopped

1 large zucchini, chopped

Freshly shredded Parmesan cheese for garnish (optional)

For pesto:

1 cup fresh basil leaves

1 teaspoon crumbled dried basil leaves

4 cloves garlic, finely minced

3 tablespoons extra-virgin olive oil

½ cup grated Parmesan cheese

Salt and freshly ground pepper to taste

Rinse dried cannellini beans and place in a large covered pot. Add chicken broth and water and bring to a boil. Uncover pot, reduce heat, and simmer until beans are tender; roughly 1 hour. Add potatoes, pasta, carrots, celery, onion, garlic, and tomato juice. Return mixture to a boil, then reduce heat and simmer uncovered for 10 minutes. Add tomatoes and zucchini, and simmer until all are tender. Process pesto ingredients in a food processor or blender until finely chopped. Remove soup from heat and stir in pesto mixture, and serve garnished with Parmesan cheese if desired.

Approx. 182 calories per serving without pesto
10g protein, 1g total fat, 0 saturated fat, 0 trans fat,
20g carbohydrates, 3mg cholesterol, 204mg sodium, 4g fiber

Approx. 254 calories per serving with pesto added
12g protein, 8g total fat, 2g saturated fat, 0 trans fat,
20g carbohydrates, 10mg cholesterol, 291mg sodium, 4g fiber

CHUNKY CHICKEN AND CABBAGE SOUP
(MAKES 4–6 SERVINGS)

4 cups low-sodium, fat-free chicken broth
2 cups water
8 ounces skinless, boneless chicken, cubed
2 medium potatoes, peeled and cubed
1 cup chopped carrots
2 bay leaves
4–6 whole peppercorns
½ teaspoon cumin
1 cup chopped celery
1 medium onion, chunked
3 cloves garlic, chopped
1 small head of cabbage, torn
2 medium tomatoes, peeled and quartered
¼ cup parsley, finely chopped
Salt and freshly ground pepper to taste
1 tablespoon plain non-fat yogurt (optional)

In a large pot, bring chicken broth, water, chicken, potatoes, carrots, bay leaves, peppercorns, and cumin to boil. Reduce heat, simmer for 30–40 minutes or until chicken is cooked. Add celery, onion, garlic, cabbage, tomatoes, and parsley; cook for additional 15 minutes or until vegetables are tender. Add salt and pepper to taste. Garnish each serving with yogurt if desired.

Approx. 143 calories per serving
15g protein, 2g total fat, <0.3g saturated fat, 0 trans fat,
21g carbohydrates, 21mg cholesterol, 50mg sodium, 3g fiber

FRENCH PISTOU SOUP
(MAKES 6 SERVINGS)

1 tablespoon extra-virgin olive oil
1 medium onion, finely chopped
½ cup dry kidney beans
2 medium potatoes, diced
1 stalk celery, chopped
2 cups chopped carrots
8 cups water
8 ounces fresh green beans cut in 1-inch pieces
1 leek, green part only, thinly sliced
2 medium tomatoes, peeled and chopped
2 small zucchini cut in 1-inch cubes
1 cup uncooked whole wheat elbow macaroni
Salt and freshly ground pepper to taste

For Pistou Mix:

3 cloves garlic
2 cups fresh basil leaves
1 tablespoon hot liquid from soup
Salt and freshly ground pepper to taste
3 tablespoons extra-virgin olive oil
Freshly grated Gruyere cheese for garnish

In large saucepan heat oil, add onion, and cook to soften. Add kidney beans, potatoes, celery, carrots, and 8 cups of water. Bring to a boil, reduce heat, and simmer covered for about 15 minutes. Add green beans, leek, tomatoes, zucchini, and pasta; cook another 10 minutes or until the vegetables are tender. Season mixture with salt and pepper to taste. Reduce heat to very low, cover to keep warm.

Make the pistou: in a food processor, finely chop garlic and basil. Add soup liquid, salt and pepper to taste, and oil. Ladle soup into individual soup bowls, then spoon in some pistou and garnish with cheese.

Approx. 248 calories per serving
10g protein, 9g total fat, 1g saturated fat, 0 trans fat,
35g carbohydrates, 0 cholesterol, 28mg sodium, 8g fiber

HEARTY BEAN SOUP
(MAKES 6–8 SERVINGS)

2 cups water
2 medium potatoes, peeled and coarsely chopped
2 large carrots, coarsely chopped
2 stalks celery, coarsely chopped
1 bay leaf
1 tablespoon fresh thyme
Salt and freshly ground pepper to taste
3 tablespoons extra-virgin olive oil
5 cloves fresh garlic, minced
1 medium onion, finely chopped
½ small hot pepper, finely chopped
5 cups low-sodium, fat-free chicken broth
4 (15-ounce) cans Great Northern beans
Grated Parmesan cheese (optional)
Chopped fresh flat leaf parsley (optional)

In a heavy pot, combine water, potato, carrots, celery, bay leaf, thyme, and salt and pepper. Bring to a boil, reduce heat, cover, and simmer until vegetables are tender. While vegetables are cooking, combine oil, garlic, onion, and hot pepper in a large skillet, and sauté until tender and lightly browned. Add 1 cup of chicken broth and beans to garlic mixture, mix together well, cover, and simmer for about 10 minutes to allow flavors to blend. Add salt and pepper to taste. Combine bean mixture and 4 cups of chicken broth, and add to vegetable pot. Stir to mix, then keep at a low simmer for about 10–15 minutes, allowing flavors to blend. Garnish with cheese and parsley, if desired.

Approx. 220 calories per serving
11g protein, 6g total fat, 0.7g saturated fat, 0 trans fat,
36g carbohydrates, 3mg cholesterol, 663mg sodium, 9g fiber

SPINACH FETA CHEESE SOUP
(MAKES 6–8 SERVINGS)

10 ounces spinach, washed under running water
6 cups low-sodium, fat-free chicken broth
¼ cup fresh cilantro, chopped
2 tablespoons extra-virgin olive oil
1 large white onion, coarsely chopped
2 medium potatoes, peeled and diced
4 cloves fresh garlic, minced
1 teaspoon ground cumin
1 (10-ounce) package frozen baby lima beans, thawed
⅓ cup couscous
6 ounces feta cheese, cut into chunks
½ teaspoon freshly ground pepper to taste
Finely chopped parsley
Lemon wedges

Cut half of the spinach leaves into thin ribbons, reserving stems, and set aside. Using a food processor or blender, combine the reserved stems and the remaining spinach with 1 cup of broth and the cilantro. Process until smooth and set aside. In a large pot, heat olive oil over medium heat, add onion, sauté until golden brown, then add potatoes, garlic, and cumin; stir to make sure potatoes are well coated. Add remaining 5 cups of broth. Reduce heat to medium and cook until potatoes are tender, roughly 15 minutes. Add ribbon spinach, spinach-cilantro puree, lima beans, couscous, and cheese. Cook until lima beans are crispy tender and cheese has melted through soup. Season soup with freshly ground pepper. Divide soup into 6–8 servings. For garnish, sprinkle parsley over soup and add a lemon wedge on the side.

Approx. 226 calories per serving
10g protein, 10g total fat, 4g saturated fat, 0 trans fat,
24g carbohydrates, 15mg cholesterol, 157mg sodium, 4g fiber

CHUNKY FISH CHOWDER WITH SAFFRON
(MAKES 6 SERVINGS)

1 pound fresh grouper fillets
1 pound fresh tuna or cod fillets
2 tablespoons extra-virgin olive oil
8–10 diced scallions
1 cup chopped celery
3 large cloves garlic, crushed
1 small yellow bell pepper, diced
1 small red bell pepper, diced
1 teaspoon turmeric
¼ teaspoon ground saffron
1¼ cup dry white wine
8 ounces bottled clam juice
4 cups water
2 bay leaves
½ teaspoon thyme
¼ teaspoon crushed red hot pepper flakes
Salt to taste
¾ cup small elbow macaroni, uncooked
2 tablespoons lemon juice
4 tablespoons chopped fresh parsley

Rinse and cut fish fillets into 1 inch cubes, refrigerate. In a large heavy-bottomed skillet, heat olive oil and sauté scallions, celery, garlic, and peppers. Add turmeric and saffron and cook a few more minutes. Stir in wine, clam juice, and water. Add in bay leaves, thyme, red pepper flakes, and salt, then bring to boil. Reduce heat and simmer for 10 minutes. Add pasta and cook until pasta is tender. Add fish and simmer for 10–15 minutes longer, until fish is cooked. Remove bay leaves. Add lemon juice, and stir to mix. Serve garnished with parsley.

Approx. 296 calories per serving
35g protein, 8g total fat, 2g saturated fat, 0 trans fat,
11g carbohydrates, 27mg cholesterol, 187mg sodium, 3g fiber

CHICKEN ESCAROLE SOUP

(MAKES 4–6 SERVINGS)

3 cups water (enough to cover chicken)
5 skinless, boneless chicken breasts, cut into chunks
1 small white onion, cut in half
⅛ cup black peppercorns
1 bay leaf
4 cloves fresh garlic, finely minced
3 cups low-sodium, fat-free chicken broth
2 medium carrots, sliced
1 celery stalk, sliced
½ head escarole, cut into 1-inch strips, stems removed
Salt and freshly ground pepper to taste
Freshly grated Parmesan cheese for garnish

In a large saucepan, combine water, chicken, onion, peppercorns, bay leaf, and garlic. Bring to a boil, reduce heat to low, cover, and simmer 1 hour or until chicken is tender. Remove chicken from broth and strain out bay leaf and peppercorns; set aside. In a separate saucepan, combine canned chicken broth with strained broth, add carrots and celery, bring to a rapid boil, reduce to low, and simmer for 10 minutes or until vegetables are crispy tender. Stir in escarole and chicken, heat through, add salt and pepper to taste, and serve. Garnish each serving with a sprinkling of grated cheese.

Approx. 153 calories per serving
28g protein, 2g total fat, <0.4g saturated fat, 0 trans fat,
4g carbohydrates, 62mg cholesterol, 129mg sodium, 5g fiber

CHILLED CUCUMBER SOUP
(MAKES 4–6 SERVINGS)

2 large English cucumbers, peeled and coarsely chopped
1 medium yellow onion, coarsely chopped
5 cups low-sodium, fat-free chicken broth
2 cups plain low-fat yogurt
2 scallions, white and green parts, finely minced
Salt to taste
Freshly ground black pepper to taste
Fresh dill, finely chopped

Combine cucumber and onion in a large saucepan; add chicken broth. Heat on high heat to rapid boil, immediately reduce to low, cover, and simmer until vegetables are just tender. Remove from heat, allow to cool slightly, then refrigerate to chill for several hours. To serve, blend in yogurt, scallions, and salt to taste. Sprinkle with freshly ground pepper and dill.

Approx. 91 calories per serving
7g protein, 3g total fat, <0.4g saturated fat, 0 trans fat,
10g carbohydrates, 4mg cholesterol, 164mg sodium, 1g fiber

EGGPLANT SOUP
(MAKES 4–6 SERVINGS)

2 tablespoons extra-virgin olive oil
2 cloves fresh garlic, minced
½ medium onion, thinly sliced and separated into rings
1 medium eggplant, peeled and cut into ½-inch cubes
½ teaspoon oregano
¼ teaspoon thyme
4 cups low-sodium, fat-free chicken broth
½ cup dry sherry
Salt and freshly ground pepper to taste
1 large tomato, sliced
10 ounces crumbled non-fat feta cheese
Freshly grated Parmesan cheese (optional)

Heat oil in large skillet over medium heat; add garlic and onion, and sauté until lightly golden. Add eggplant, oregano, and thyme; continue cooking until eggplant browns slightly, stirring constantly. Reduce heat to low, add broth, cover, and simmer for roughly 5 minutes. Add sherry, cover, and continue to simmer for another 2–3 minutes. Stir in salt and pepper to taste if needed, and remove from heat. Allow to cool slightly. Preheat broiler, and pour slightly cooled soup into an oven-safe bowl. Top soup with tomato slices and feta cheese, place soup under broiler, and heat until feta melts into soup. Garnish with grated Parmesan cheese if desired, and broil until cheese is browned.

Approx. 146 calories per serving
9g protein, 5g total fat, <1g saturated fat, 0 trans fat,
10g carbohydrates, 3mg cholesterol, 538mg sodium, 2g fiber

PASTA e FAGIOLI SOUP
(MAKES 14 1-CUP SERVINGS)

2 tablespoons extra-virgin olive oil
6 cloves fresh garlic, minced
1½ cups chopped carrot
1½ cups chopped celery
1½ cups chopped white onion
3 cups water
3 (14.5-ounce) cans low-sodium, fat-free chicken broth
3 teaspoons dried parsley
1½ teaspoons dried mixed Italian seasoning
¼ teaspoon dried hot red pepper flakes
1 (14.5-ounce) can diced tomatoes with liquid
½ cup dried ditalini pasta
½ cup dried kidney beans
½ cup dried cannellini beans
Salt and freshly ground black pepper to taste
Freshly grated Parmesan cheese for garnish

In a large skillet, add oil and sauté garlic, carrots, celery, and onions. Transfer to a large heavy-bottomed pot; add water, broth, parsley, Italian seasoning, pepper flakes, tomatoes, pasta, beans, and salt and pepper to taste. Bring soup to a boil, cover, and reduce to a simmer for about 2–3 hours or until beans are soft. Serve with a sprinkling of grated Parmesan cheese.

Approx. 150 calories per 1 cup serving
6g protein, 0.5g total fat, 0 saturated fat, <0.1g trans fat,
18g carbohydrates, 0 cholesterol, 5mg sodium, 4g fiber

MOM'S CHICKEN SOUP
(MAKES 8–10 SERVINGS)

3 (5–6-ounce) skinless, boneless chicken breasts cut into 1-inch cubes
2 cups water
4 garlic cloves, chopped
3 large carrots, cut into small chunks
4–6 celery stalks, cut into small chunks
1 medium yellow onion, cut into chunks
8 cups fat-free, low-sodium chicken broth
½ cup dry orzo
1 tablespoon extra-virgin olive oil
Freshly ground pepper to taste
Tabasco sauce if desired

In a large pot, add chicken cubes, water, and garlic. Bring to a boil, cover, and reduce heat to a simmer. Simmer for about 10 minutes. Add carrots, celery, and onions, and cook for an additional 5–10 minutes. Add chicken broth, orzo, olive oil, and pepper to taste. Continue to simmer on low heat, covered, until orzo is soft. Serve with a drizzle of Tabasco sauce if desired.

Approx. 131 calories per serving
16g protein, 3g total fat, 0.4g saturated fat, 0 trans fat,
12g carbohydrates, 29mg cholesterol, 513mg sodium, 1g fiber

POTATO LEEK SOUP WITH SMOKED SALMON
(MAKES 8 SERVINGS)

1 tablespoon extra-virgin olive oil
2 tablespoons trans fat–free canola/olive oil spread
2 large leeks, white and light green parts only, cut in half lengthwise and
    thinly sliced
2 medium fennel bulbs, trimmed and chopped
1 teaspoon fennel seeds
6 cups low-sodium, low-fat chicken broth
2 pounds red potatoes, peeled and cubed (2-inch cubes)
2 ounces thinly sliced nova lox, cut into pieces
Salt and freshly ground pepper to taste
Freshly chopped chives for garnish

In a heavy pan heat olive oil over medium-high heat; add spread and allow to melt. Add leeks, fennel, and fennel seeds, and sauté until translucent (about 7 minutes). Add broth and potatoes to skillet and bring to a boil. Reduce to medium-low heat and simmer until potatoes are tender (about 20–25 minutes). Transfer soup in batches to a blender and puree. Return to pot to warm on low heat. When soup is warm, add smoked salmon pieces, salt and pepper to taste, and serve, garnished with fresh-chopped chives.

Approx. 144 calories per serving
10g protein, 10g total fat, 0.89g saturated fat, 0 trans fat,
23g carbohydrates, 0 cholesterol, 92mg sodium, 4g fiber

Pizza, Pizza Sauces, and Pizza Crusts

In the Mediterranean regions, a pizza made at home is a well-balanced modern meal, made from complex carbohydrate pizza dough, fresh vegetables, small amounts of animal protein, and monounsaturated fat in the form of extra-virgin olive oil. In contrast, the fast food pizza made in the United States is loaded with saturated fat, trans fats, refined sugar, and sodium.

For healthy, quick, and easy pizzas, just top Toufayan's round whole grain wraps or Flat Out's oval, light whole grain wraps (both are trans fat–free and make great quick pizza crusts) with your favorite pizza ingredients and bake in the oven at 350 degrees for about 5 minutes or until cheese melts and edges of wrap become crispy.

SMOKED SALMON AND MOZZARELLA CHEESE PIZZA
(MAKES AN 8-INCH PERSONAL PIZZA)

1 flat wrap
1 tablespoon fresh Basil Pesto Sauce (page 357) or a market-fresh basil pesto
4 slices of smoked nova (about 2 ounces)
2 tablespoons coarsely chopped red onion
¼ cup shredded part-skim mozzarella cheese
Dried oregano flakes to sprinkle

Preheat oven to 350 degrees. Place wrap on a baking sheet and spread pesto sauce lightly over surface of wrap. Arrange salmon over pesto and scatter on onions and cheese. Sprinkle with oregano and bake at 350 degrees until cheese melts and begins to bubble. Remove from oven and serve.

Approx. 325 calories per pizza
28g protein, 16g total fat, 3g saturated fat, 0 trans fat,
17g carbohydrates, 30mg cholesterol, 145mg sodium, 8g fiber

ASSORTED MUSHROOM AND SWISS CHEESE PIZZA
(MAKES AN 8-INCH PERSONAL PIZZA)

1 flat wrap
1 tablespoon extra-virgin olive oil
½ cup sliced assorted mushrooms
2 tablespoons chopped scallions, white and green parts
2 teaspoons fresh garlic paste
Freshly ground pepper to taste
1 ounce shredded light Swiss cheese
1 tablespoon dried thyme, finely crushed

Preheat oven to 350 degrees. Place wrap on a baking sheet and set aside. Heat a small amount of oil in a heavy-bottomed skillet. Add mushrooms, scallions, garlic paste, and pepper. Sauté for 2–3 minutes, stirring often, until mushrooms and scallions soften. Remove from heat and spread mixture out evenly over wrap. Distribute cheese over mushroom mixture and sprinkle on thyme. Place in oven and bake at 350 degrees until cheese melts. Remove from oven and serve.

Approx. 262 calories per pizza
24g protein, 8g total fat, 4g saturated fat, 0 trans fat,
18g carbohydrates, 20mg cholesterol, 607mg sodium, 8g fiber

BABY SHRIMP AND MOZZARELLA CHEESE PIZZA
(MAKES AN 8-INCH PERSONAL PIZZA)

1 flat wrap
1 tablespoon fresh Basil Pesto Sauce (page 357) or a market-fresh basil pesto
½ cup cooked baby salad shrimp, defrosted (if frozen) and well drained
4 small pitted black olives, drained and sliced
¼ cup shredded part-skim mozzarella cheese
Dried chives to sprinkle

Preheat oven to 350 degrees. Place wrap on a baking sheet and spread pesto evenly over surface of wrap. Scatter well-drained shrimp over pesto, add olives, and top with cheese. Sprinkle chives over cheese and bake at 350 degrees until cheese melts and begins to bubble. Remove from oven and serve.

Approx. 371 calories per pizza
37g protein, 18g total fat, 5g saturated fat, 0 trans fat,
18g carbohydrates, 70mg cholesterol, 121mg sodium, 9g fiber

FRESH BASIL AND MOZZARELLA CHEESE PIZZA
(MAKES AN 8-INCH PERSONAL PIZZA)

1 flat wrap
1 teaspoon finely minced garlic
¼ cup fresh Traditional Pizza Sauce (page 127) or a market sauce like Dei
  Fratelli
¼ cup shredded part-skim mozzarella cheese
4 slices fresh tomato
4–6 fresh whole basil leaves

Preheat oven to 350 degrees. Place wrap on a baking sheet. Stir garlic into tomato sauce and spread evenly over wrap. Top sauce first with cheese then tomatoes and basil leaves. Bake at 350 degrees until cheese melts. Remove from oven and serve.

Approx. 270 calories per pizza
23g protein, 9g total fat, 4g saturated fat, 0 trans fat,
25g carbohydrates, 15mg cholesterol, 888mg sodium, 10g fiber

TOMATO, EGGPLANT, AND BASIL PIZZA

(MAKES AN 8-SLICE, 15-INCH PIZZA)

Crispy Thin Whole Wheat Pizza Dough (page 130)
1 large eggplant
6 garlic cloves, minced
2 tablespoons extra-virgin olive oil
5 medium tomatoes, seeded and chopped
3 tablespoons chopped fresh basil
Pinch of hot pepper flakes
3 cups crumbled non-fat feta cheese
Salt and freshly ground black pepper to taste
⅓ cup freshly grated Parmesan cheese
Fresh rosemary, finely chopped (optional)

Preheat oven to 425 degrees. Follow directions for pizza dough and roll out to a 12–15-inch round. Place pizza round on scantly oiled pizza pan. Cut eggplant in half the long way, slashing down the middle but not through the skin. Place on pan and bake for 20–30 minutes. Skin should be shriveled and eggplant tender. Remove to a plate and reserve; when cooled, slice crosswise into thin slices. Sauté garlic in 1 tablespoon of olive oil over low heat until softened. Add tomatoes, basil, and hot pepper flakes. Brush pizza dough lightly with ½ teaspoon olive oil, top with tomato mixture, then feta cheese, and arrange eggplant slices in a pinwheel pattern, slightly overlapping the slices. Season pizza with salt and pepper and drizzle remaining olive oil over eggplant. Bake at 425 degrees for 10–15 minutes until pizza crust is crisp. Garnish top of pizza with Parmesan cheese and rosemary if desired.

Approx. 166 calories per slice
20g protein, 4g total fat, <0.5g saturated fat, 0 trans fat,
21g carbohydrates, 0 cholesterol, 185mg sodium, 1g fiber

PIZZA MARGHERITA
(MAKES AN 8-SLICE, 15-INCH PIZZA)

Thin Crust Pizza Dough (page 132)
4 Roma tomatoes, thinly sliced
Salt and freshly ground pepper to taste
½ cup yellow sweet pepper, thinly sliced
¾ cup shredded part-skim mozzarella cheese, about 3 ounces
4–5 snipped fresh basil leaves
¼ cup freshly grated Parmesan cheese
1 tablespoon extra-virgin olive oil

Preheat oven to 450 degrees. Follow directions for pizza dough and roll out to a 12–15-inch round. Place dough on a scantly oiled pizza pan. Spread tomatoes on rolled-out dough almost to the edge of the crust. Sprinkle with salt and pepper to taste. Top tomatoes with yellow peppers, mozzarella cheese, basil, and Parmesan cheese, and drizzle olive oil over the top. Bake at 450 degrees for 8–10 minutes or until crust is crisp and cheeses are melted.

Approx. 202 calories per slice
11g protein, 7g total fat, 3g saturated fat, 0 trans fat,
28g carbohydrates, 7mg cholesterol, 375mg sodium, 1g fiber

SPICY SWEET PEPPER PIZZA
(MAKES AN 8-SLICE, 15-INCH PIZZA)

Whole Wheat Pizza Dough (page 131)
1 tablespoon extra-virgin olive oil
3 large red bell peppers, seeded and thinly sliced
3 large yellow bell peppers, seeded and thinly sliced
2 cloves garlic, minced
1 tablespoon chopped fresh thyme
Salt and freshly ground pepper to taste
Hot pepper flakes to taste
1 cup shredded part-skim mozzarella cheese

Preheat oven to 500 degrees. Follow directions for pizza dough and roll out to 12–15-inch round. Place dough on scantly oiled pizza pan. Heat oil in heavy-bottomed pan and sauté the peppers and garlic, about 10 minutes until soft. Stir in thyme, salt and pepper to taste, and red pepper flakes. Spread pepper mixture over pizza dough, sprinkle cheese over pepper mixture, and bake for 20–25 minutes until crust is crisp and cheese has melted.

Approx. 209 calories per slice
9g protein, 7g total fat, 3g saturated fat, 0 trans fat,
25g carbohydrates, 7mg cholesterol, 78mg sodium, 4g fiber

WILD MUSHROOM PIZZA
(MAKES AN 8-SLICE, 15-INCH PIZZA)

Thin Crust Pizza Dough (page 132)
3 ounces dried porcine mushrooms
1 quart warm water
2 tablespoons extra-virgin olive oil
4 cloves garlic, finely minced
1 cup fresh button mushrooms, cleaned and thinly sliced
1 cup fresh shiitake or other wild mushroom
4 tablespoons white wine
1 tablespoon low-sodium soy sauce
½ teaspoon dried thyme
½ teaspoon dried rosemary
Salt and freshly ground pepper to taste
3 tablespoons chopped fresh parsley
8 ounces shredded smoked provolone cheese

Preheat oven to 425 degrees. Follow directions for pizza dough; when ready, roll it out to a 15-inch round. Place on scantly oiled pizza pan. Soak the dried mushrooms in warm water for 30 minutes. After soaking, squeeze excess liquid from mushrooms and chop coarsely. Strain soaking water through a cheesecloth and set aside. Heat 1 tablespoon of olive oil over medium heat in a heavy-bottomed skillet and add half of the garlic. Sauté garlic, stirring often until it becomes golden. Add both dried and fresh mushrooms, sauté for about 5 minutes until they begin to release their liquid, and then add wine and soy sauce. Continue to sauté until wine evaporates. Add soaking liquid to mushrooms, thyme, rosemary, remaining garlic, and salt and pepper to taste. Increase heat; continue cooking and stirring until most of the liquid has evaporated and mushrooms have become glazed. Add parsley and remove from heat. Brush pizza dough with remaining olive oil. Evenly spread cheese over crust. Spread mushroom mixture over cheese and bake for roughly 8–10 minutes, until crust is crisp and cheese is melted.

Approx. 208 calories per slice
9g protein, 10g total fat, 0.5g saturated fat, 0 trans fat,
22g carbohydrates, 0 cholesterol, 351mg sodium, 2g fiber

SUNDRIED TOMATO AND ANCHOVY PIZZA
(MAKES AN 8-SLICE, 15-INCH PIZZA)

Crispy Thin Whole Wheat Pizza Dough (page 130)
1 red onion, thinly sliced
8 sundried tomatoes in oil, chopped
1 tablespoon basil leaves, broken in pieces
1 can (2 ounces) anchovy fillets, chopped, oil reserved
1 clove garlic, minced
1 cup fresh part-skim mozzarella cheese, shredded
Salt and freshly ground pepper to taste
Finely chopped fresh parsley for garnish (optional)

Preheat oven to 425 degrees. Follow directions for pizza dough; when ready, roll out to 15-inch round. Place on scantly oiled pizza pan. Top pizza crust dough with onions, sundried tomatoes, basil, anchovies, garlic, and fresh mozzarella. Salt and pepper to taste and bake at 425 degrees until crust is crisp and cheese is melted. Garnish with parsley if desired.

Approx. 137 calories per slice
6g protein, 5g total fat, 3g saturated fat, 0 trans fat,
18g carbohydrates, 10mg cholesterol, 119mg sodium, 1g fiber

Pizza Sauces

TRADITIONAL PIZZA SAUCE
(MAKES ENOUGH FOR A 15-INCH CRUST)

2 tablespoons extra-virgin olive oil
3 cloves garlic, peeled and sliced
5 medium tomatoes, seeded and chopped
2 sprigs fresh rosemary
Salt and freshly ground pepper to taste
Pinch of sugar

In a heavy skillet over medium-high heat, add oil and garlic and cook until soft. Add tomatoes, herbs, salt and pepper, and sugar; raise heat slightly and cook rapidly, stirring often until juices thicken (about 15–20 minutes). Put sauce through a food mill, letting pulp pass through. If sauce is too thin, return to low heat and cook until desired consistency.

Approx. 63 calories per serving, based on a 2-inch slice
1g protein, 4g total fat, <0.5g saturated fat, 0 trans fat,
4g carbohydrates, 0 cholesterol, 390mg sodium, 1g fiber

FIERY TOMATO AND BASIL PIZZA SAUCE
(MAKES ENOUGH FOR A 15-INCH CRUST)

1 tablespoon extra-virgin olive oil
4 cloves garlic, chopped
5 medium tomatoes, seeded and chopped
3 tablespoons fresh chopped basil
Salt and freshly ground pepper to taste
Pinch of sugar
¼ teaspoon hot pepper flakes

In skillet, heat olive oil over medium-high heat and sauté garlic. Add tomatoes, cook, and stir for about 5 minutes. Combine basil, salt and pepper, sugar, and hot pepper, and add to tomato mixture.

Approx. 38 calories per serving, based on a 2-inch slice
1g protein, 2g total fat, <0.5g saturated fat, 0 trans fat,
3g carbohydrates, 0 cholesterol, 7mg sodium, 1g fiber

SPICY GARLIC, OLIVE OIL,
AND SUNDRIED TOMATO PIZZA SAUCE
(MAKES ENOUGH FOR A 12-INCH CRUST)

¼ cup extra-virgin olive oil
4 cloves garlic, minced
¼ teaspoon red hot pepper flakes
6 jumbo pitted black olives, diced
8 sundried tomatoes in oil, drained and diced
Salt and freshly ground pepper to taste

In a medium-sized skillet, heat olive oil over medium-high heat, add garlic, and sauté until translucent. Add hot pepper flakes, olives, and sundried tomato, and salt and pepper to taste; simmer over very low heat for 3–5 minutes.

Approx. 79 calories per slice, based on a 2-inch slice
0 protein, 9g total fat, 1g saturated fat, 0 trans fat,
1g carbohydrates, 0 cholesterol, 42mg sodium, 0 fiber

EASY PIZZA SAUCE
(MAKES 1 QUART OF SAUCE)

1 teaspoon crumbled dried basil
½ teaspoon crumbled dried oregano
¼ teaspoon crumbled dried marjoram
¼ cup dry white wine
2 cloves garlic, finely chopped
1 tablespoon extra-virgin olive oil
1½ cups chopped crushed plum tomato
2 tablespoons tomato paste
Salt and freshly ground black pepper to taste

Add herbs to wine and marinate for 15 minutes. Meanwhile, over medium heat, sauté garlic in olive oil until soft but not brown. Add tomatoes, tomato paste, and herb/wine mixture. Cover and simmer for about 20 minutes. Remove from stove, put into a blender, and puree until smooth. Return to skillet uncovered and continue to simmer until sauce thickens slightly.

Approx. 19 calories per ¼ cup
0.4g protein, 1g total fat, 0 saturated fat, 0 trans fat,
2g carbohydrates, 0 cholesterol, 102mg sodium, 0.23g fiber

Pizza Crusts

CRISPY THIN WHOLE WHEAT PIZZA DOUGH
(MAKES AN 8-SLICE, 15-INCH CRUST)

⅔ cup all-purpose unbleached flour
1 package active dry yeast
⅛ teaspoon salt
½ cup warm water
1 teaspoon extra-virgin olive oil
½ cup whole wheat flour
4 tablespoons all-purpose flour
Non-stick olive oil cooking spray

In a mixing bowl combine all-purpose flour, yeast, and salt. Add water and oil and beat on high speed for about 2–3 minutes. Use a wooden spoon to stir in whole wheat flour. Transfer mixture to a lightly floured surface and knead in 1–2 additional tablespoons of all-purpose flour as you form mixture into a ball that is slightly stiff, yet still smooth and elastic. Put dough into a clean bowl, cover, and place in a warm area for about 10 minutes. Spray a pizza pan lightly with oil spray. Roll out dough on a lightly floured surface into a 15-inch round, place on pizza pan, and top with sauce and ingredients of choice. Bake at 425 degrees for about 10 minutes, or until crust is crispy.

Approx. 76 calories per slice, crust only
2g protein, 0.5g total fat, 0.5g saturated fat, 0 trans fat,
16g carbohydrates, 0 cholesterol, 35mg sodium, 1g fiber

WHOLE WHEAT PIZZA DOUGH
(MAKES AN 8-SLICE, 15-INCH CRUST)

2½ teaspoons active dry yeast
1½ teaspoon low-calorie baking sweetener
1 teaspoon salt
2 tablespoons extra-virgin olive oil
½ cup lukewarm water
2 cups whole wheat flour
3–4 tablespoons extra flour for kneading

In a bowl, mix together yeast, sweetener, salt, oil, and water. Set aside for 10 minutes; the mixture will become cloudy and thick. When this happens, make a well in the center of the dough. Add yeast mixture and gradually fold it into the flour, adding more lukewarm water if needed. Knead dough until it becomes smooth, then place dough in a lightly oiled bowl and cover with a clean cloth. Place dough in a warm area for about 45 minutes or until it doubles its size. Roll out dough on a lightly floured surface into a 15-inch round, place on pizza pan, and top with sauce and ingredients of choice. Bake at 500 degrees until crust is crispy.

Approx. 142 calories per slice, crust only
5g protein, 3g total fat, <0.5g saturated fat, 0 trans fat,
22g carbohydrates, 0 cholesterol, 3mg sodium, 4g fiber

THIN CRUST PIZZA DOUGH
(MAKES AN 8-SLICE, 15-INCH CRUST)

1⅔ cups unbleached all-purpose flour
½ teaspoon salt
1 package dry active yeast
2 tablespoons extra-virgin olive oil
½ cup warm water
Olive oil to lightly coat pan

Put flour, salt, and yeast in a large bowl and mix with a wooden spoon. Make a well in the center and add oil and water. Gradually work in flour from the sides of the bowl as the mixture becomes smooth, pliable, soft dough. If too sticky, sprinkle a little more flour into the mixture, but don't make the dough dry. Transfer dough to a lightly floured surface and knead for about 10 minutes; add very small amounts of flour if needed until dough becomes smooth and elastic. Rub a small amount of oil over the surface of the dough, then return it to a clean bowl, cover it with a cloth, and place it in a warm area for about 1 hour or until dough doubles in size. Remove dough to a lightly floured surface, knead for an additional 2 minutes, then roll out into a 15-inch round. Place on pizza pan and top with sauce and ingredients of choice. Bake at 425 degrees until crust is crispy.

Approx. 115 calories per slice, crust only
2g protein, 3g total fat, <0.5g saturated fat, 0 trans fat,
18g carbohydrates, 0 cholesterol, 144mg sodium, 0 fiber

BREAD MACHINE WHOLE GRAIN THIN CRUST PIZZA DOUGH
(MAKES 2 4-SLICE, 12-INCH CRUSTS)

1 cup water (room temperature)
2 tablespoons canola oil
1 tablespoon low-calorie baking sweetener
½ teaspoon salt (optional) or ½ teaspoon sodium-free salt substitute
1 cup whole grain flour
1½ cups bread flour
2¼ teaspoons active dry yeast

Add water, oil, sweetener, salt, both flours, and yeast to bread machine canister, in that order. Set bread machine program to dough setting. When the machine turns off, remove dough ball from canister and place on a lightly floured flat surface. Divide ball in half and press or roll out each half to fit a 12-inch pizza pan or stone. Curl up edges of dough and prick the surface of the dough with a fork. Place pan or stone on the middle rack of an oven preheated to 400 degrees for about 10–12 minutes or until the crust turns a light golden brown. Remove baked crust from oven, top with sauce and ingredients of choice, and return to bake for additional 10–15 minutes or until cheese has melted.

Approx. 54 calories per 3-inch-wide slice, crust only
2g protein, 1g total fat, 0.75g saturated fat, 0 trans fat,
9g carbohydrates, 0 cholesterol, 49mg sodium, 1g fiber

Omelets and Frittatas

CHEESY APPLE RAISIN CINNAMON OMELET
(MAKES 4 SERVINGS)

1 medium sweet apple (Fiji, Fuji, or Golden Delicious), peeled, cored, and
  sliced
1 tablespoon extra-virgin olive oil
2 tablespoons seedless black raisins
1 cup egg substitute or 1 cup egg whites or 4 whole eggs
2 tablespoons crumbled blue cheese
2 tablespoons freshly shredded Parmesan cheese
Salt and freshly ground pepper to taste
⅛ teaspoon cinnamon

Sauté apples in ½ tablespoon of olive oil until crispy tender; add raisins, then immediately remove apple mixture from pan and transfer to a bowl. Combine eggs, cheeses, and salt and pepper, and mix well. Heat remaining oil in an omelet pan; cook ¼ of egg mixture at a time, on low heat, lifting edges to allow uncooked portion to flow under and cook. Repeat process 4 times for each serving. Arrange ¼ apple mixture onto one half of cooked egg. Fold in half and sprinkle top with cinnamon. Serve as a breakfast omelet or a dessert.

Approx. 116 calories per omelet, using egg substitute
7g protein, 8g total fat, 1g saturated fat, 0 trans fat,
9g carbohydrates, 4mg cholesterol, 206mg sodium, 0 fiber

Approx. 111 calories per omelet, using egg whites
6g protein, 8g total fat, 1g saturated fat, 0 trans fat,
8g carbohydrates, 4mg cholesterol, 166mg sodium, 0 fiber

Approx. 166 calories, using fresh whole eggs
6g protein, 13g total fat, 3g saturated fat, 0 trans fat,
8g carbohydrates, 244mg cholesterol, 161mg sodium, 0 fiber

MIXED VEGETABLE FRITTATA
(MAKES 4 SERVINGS)

10 large fresh asparagus spears
1½ cups egg substitute or 1½ cups egg whites or 6 whole eggs
¾ cup low-fat cottage cheese
2 teaspoons spicy brown mustard
¼ teaspoon crushed dried tarragon
¼ teaspoon marjoram
Salt and freshly ground pepper to taste
½ teaspoon extra-virgin olive oil
1 cup sliced fresh mushrooms
½ cup diced onions
¼ cup chopped seeded tomatoes for garnish

Boil asparagus for 8–10 minutes until crispy tender. Drain. Cut all but three spears into 1-inch pieces. Set aside. In a bowl mix together egg, cottage cheese, mustard, tarragon, marjoram, and salt and pepper. Set aside. Heat olive oil in a large oven-safe skillet, and sauté mushrooms and onions until tender. Stir in asparagus pieces, pour egg mixture over top, and cook an additional 5 minutes over low heat until it bubbles and begins to set. Arrange remaining three uncut asparagus on top of mixture. Place skillet in oven and bake uncovered at 400 degrees for 10 minutes or until frittata sets. Remove from heat. Sprinkle with tomatoes and serve.

Approx. 169 calories per serving, using egg substitute
17g protein, 1g total fat, <0.5g saturated fat, 0 trans fat,
7g carbohydrates, 321mg cholesterol, 369mg sodium, 2g fiber

Approx. 164 calories per serving, using egg whites
16g protein, 1g total fat, <0.5g saturated fat, 0 trans fat,
6g carbohydrates, 321mg cholesterol, 329mg sodium, 2g fiber

Approx. 216 calories per serving, using fresh whole eggs
18g protein, 11g total fat, 3.5g saturated fat, 0 trans fat,
7g carbohydrates, 561mg cholesterol, 324mg sodium, 2g fiber

SPANISH OMELET
(MAKES 6 MAIN-COURSE SERVINGS)

2 tablespoons extra-virgin olive oil
6 whole scallions, coarsely chopped
4 garlic cloves, thinly sliced
1 green bell pepper, seeded and thinly sliced
1 red bell pepper, seeded and thinly sliced
1 medium zucchini, diced
3 ripe tomatoes, peeled and cut into wedges
Salt and freshly ground pepper to taste
¼ teaspoon cayenne pepper to taste
¾ teaspoon ground cumin
½ teaspoon ground coriander
½ teaspoon ground cinnamon
4 tablespoons chopped fresh parsley
3 cups egg substitute or 3 cups egg whites or 12 large eggs
¼ pound crumbled fresh low-fat goat cheese

Heat 2 tablespoons olive oil in an oven-safe skillet and gently sauté onions and garlic for about 5 minutes, until they begin to soften. Add the green and red peppers, zucchini, and tomatoes, raise heat slightly, and continue sautéing another 5–10 minutes until the vegetables have softened and most of the juice is absorbed. Add salt and pepper to taste. Set aside at room temperature. In a large bowl combine the herbs with the eggs, and mix with a fork just enough to break up the yolks. Lift the vegetables out of the skillet with a slotted spoon and combine with eggs. Return the skillet to medium heat, adding more oil if necessary. When the oil is hot add the eggs and vegetable mixture and cook for 2–3 minutes, lifting the edges with a spatula to allow uncooked eggs to run under cooked ones. Crumble cheese over the top of the omelet and transfer skillet to a 400-degree oven to finish cooking for about 15–20 minutes or until omelet is set and the cheese is melted. Can also be served as a light supper.

Approx. 125 calories per serving, using egg substitute
10g protein, 9g total fat, 1g saturated fat, 0 trans fat,
6g carbohydrates, 8mg cholesterol, 190mg sodium, 1g fiber

Approx. 121 calories per serving, using egg whites
9g protein, 9g total fat, 1g saturated fat, 0 trans fat,
5g carbohydrates, 8mg cholesterol, 150mg sodium, 1g fiber

Approx. 176 calories per serving, using fresh whole eggs
11g protein, 19g total fat, 3g saturated fat, 0 trans fat,
6g carbohydrates, 248mg cholesterol, 145mg sodium, 1g fiber

BROCCOLI AND CHEESE FRITTATA
(MAKES 6 MAIN COURSE SERVINGS)

3 cups broccoli florets
1 tablespoon extra-virgin olive oil
½ cup finely chopped onion
½ cup chopped red bell pepper
2 cloves garlic, minced
1 cup shredded mozzarella cheese
Dash of crushed red hot pepper flakes
1½ cups egg substitute or 1½ cups egg whites or 6 large eggs

Steam broccoli until crispy tender and remove from heat. In a large skillet over medium-high heat add olive oil, and sauté onions, bell peppers, and garlic until vegetables are soft (about 5 minutes). Add broccoli, and cook about 2 minutes longer. Transfer vegetable mixture to a bowl, then add cheese and crushed hot peppers. If using whole eggs, beat in a separate bowl until blended. Stir eggs into vegetable mixture and pour into a round cake pan lightly sprayed with olive oil spray. Bake in 325-degree oven until eggs are set, about 30 minutes. Serve hot or at room temperature.

Approx. 121 calories per serving, using egg substitute
12g protein, 8g total fat, 4g saturated fat, 0 trans fat,
5g carbohydrates, 10mg cholesterol, 209mg sodium, 0 fiber

Approx. 116 calories per serving, using egg whites
11g protein, 8g total fat, 4g saturated fat, 0 trans fat,
4g carbohydrates, 10mg cholesterol, 169mg sodium, 0 fiber

Approx. 166 calories per serving, using fresh whole eggs
12g protein, 18g total fat, 8g saturated fat, 0 trans fat,
5g carbohydrates, 197mg cholesterol, 172mg sodium, 1g fiber

ZUCCHINI FRITTATA
(MAKES 6 SERVINGS)

1½ tablespoons extra-virgin olive oil
1 medium yellow onion, chopped
2 cloves garlic, minced
3 small zucchini, sliced ¼-inch thick
Salt and freshly ground pepper to taste
2 tablespoons minced fresh basil leaves
2 cups egg substitute or 2 cups egg whites or 8 large eggs
½ cup (2 ounces) freshly grated Parmesan cheese

In a skillet over medium-low heat, add oil, and sauté onions and garlic until soft and lightly browned. Add zucchini and salt and pepper to onion/garlic mixture and cook another 5–8 minutes. Remove from heat and set aside. In a bowl, add basil and eggs (beat eggs if using whole eggs) to zucchini mixture. Stir mixture to blend and pour egg mixture into a lightly greased round cake pan. Bake in oven at 325 degrees until eggs set. Remove from oven, sprinkle cheese over top of frittata, and place under broiler for 2–3 minutes until cheese is golden brown. Remove from oven and serve immediately. Can be served as a light supper.

Approx. 126 calories per serving, using egg substitute
12g protein, 6g total fat, 2g saturated fat, 0 trans fat,
11g carbohydrates, 7mg cholesterol, 312mg sodium, 1g fiber

Approx. 121 calories per serving, using egg whites
11g protein, 6g total fat, 2g saturated fat, 0 trans fat,
4g carbohydrates, 7mg cholesterol, 244mg sodium, 1g fiber

Approx. 161 calories per serving, using whole eggs
10g protein, 10g total fat, 4g saturated fat, 0 trans fat,
4g carbohydrates, 195mg cholesterol, 242mg sodium, 1g fiber

VEGETABLE OMELET WITH PESTO
(MAKES 6 SERVINGS)

½ teaspoons extra-virgin olive oil
1 cup sliced white mushrooms
⅔ medium red onion, diced
½ cup fresh peas, cooked and drained
2 whole carrots, cleaned, cut julienne style, cooked, and drained
   (Option: substitute other vegetables if desired)
2 tablespoons Basil Pesto Sauce (page 357) or a market-fresh pesto sauce
Olive oil cooking spray
3 cups egg substitute or 3 cups egg whites or 12 whole fresh eggs
¼ cup water
¼ teaspoon salt
¼ teaspoon pepper
6 sprigs basil for garnish

In a medium skillet heat olive oil and sauté mushrooms and onions, then remove from heat. Mix all other vegetables with onions and mix in prepared pesto. Spray a non-stick 15x10x1-inch baking pan with olive oil spray and set aside. In a mixing bowl combine egg with water and salt and pepper. Beat until frothy. Pour egg mixture into pan, and bake uncovered at 400 degrees for about 8 minutes or until mixture is set. Cut baked eggs into 6 (5-inch) squares and remove squares from pan. Spoon ¼ cup of vegetable mixture on half of each omelet square, fold over, and garnish with basil sprigs.

Approx. 103 calories per serving, using egg substitute
7g protein, 5g total fat, 0.7g saturated fat, 0 trans fat,
6g carbohydrates, 0 cholesterol, 137mg sodium, 2g fiber

Approx. 83 calories per serving, using egg white
7g protein, 5g total fat, 0.7g saturated fat, 0 trans fat,
6g carbohydrates, 0 cholesterol, 97mg sodium, 2g fiber

Approx. 161 calories per serving, using whole eggs
7g protein, 15g total fat, 4g saturated fat, 0 trans fat,
6g carbohydrates, 34mg cholesterol, 92mg sodium, 2g fiber

Pancakes

STRAWBERRY BUTTERMILK PANCAKES
(MAKES 12 PANCAKES)

2 cups whole grain pastry flour
1 teaspoon baking powder
¼ teaspoon baking soda
¼ teaspoon salt (optional)
2 cups low-fat buttermilk
½ cup egg substitute
1 cup sliced fresh strawberries
Canola oil cooking spray
Sliced strawberries or other fruit as garnish (optional)
Sugar-free syrup

In a mixing bowl whisk together flour, baking powder, baking soda, and salt, then make a well in the center of the mixture. In a separate bowl combine the buttermilk and eggs, and whisk to blend. Pour milk mixture into the well and fold in flour with a spatula until mixture is smooth. Gently fold in strawberries and allow batter to stand for 5 minutes. In the meantime, spray a griddle with cooking spray and heat over medium heat. Drop a few droplets of water onto heated griddle. When water droplets bead, griddle is hot enough. Pour 2 tablespoons of batter onto griddle for each pancake. Cook pancakes until the surface of pancake begins to bubble and the edges turn golden brown (about 3 minutes). Flip pancake over and cook until other side is golden brown. Repeat this process until all the batter is gone. Keep cooked pancakes on a warm platter or in a low-heat oven (175 degrees) while preparing the other pancakes. Serve warm, garnished with sliced strawberries, sugar-free syrup, or low-sugar fruit jams if desired.

Approx. 53 calories per pancake
4g protein, < 0.5g total fat, 0 saturated fat, 0 trans fat,
15g carbohydrates, 1mg cholesterol, 124mg sodium, 2g fiber

BANANA BUTTERMILK PANCAKES
(MAKES 12 PANCAKES)

2 cups whole grain pastry flour
1 teaspoon baking powder
¼ teaspoon baking soda
¼ teaspoon salt (optional)
2 cups low-fat buttermilk
½ cup egg substitute
1 cup mashed ripe banana
Canola oil cooking spray
Sliced banana or sugar-free or low-sugar fruit jams as garnish (optional)
Sugar-free syrup

In a mixing bowl whisk together flour, baking powder, baking soda, and salt, then make a well in the center of the mixture. In a separate bowl combine the buttermilk and eggs and whisk to blend. Pour milk mixture into well and fold in flour with a spatula until mixture is smooth. Gently fold in bananas and allow batter to stand for 5 minutes. In the meantime, spray a griddle with cooking spray and heat over medium heat. Drop a few droplets of water onto heated griddle. When water droplets bead, griddle is hot enough. Pour 2 tablespoons of batter onto griddle for each pancake. Cook pancakes until the surface of pancake begins to bubble and the edges turn golden brown (about 3 minutes). Flip pancake over and cook until other side is golden brown. Repeat this process until all the batter is gone. Keep cooked pancakes on a warm platter or in a low-heat oven (175 degrees) while preparing the other pancakes. Serve warm, garnished with sliced bananas, sugar-free syrup, or low-sugar fruit jams if desired.

Approx. 66 calories per pancake
4g protein, <0.5g total fat, 0 saturated fat, 0 trans fat,
18g carbohydrates, 1mg cholesterol, 124mg sodium, 2g fiber

MULTIGRAIN NUTTY BLUEBERRY PANCAKES
(MAKES 6 PANCAKES)

¾ cup multigrain pancake flour
½ cup + 2 tablespoons skim milk
1 tablespoon canola oil
¼ cup blueberries (either fresh or frozen)
⅛ cup chopped walnuts
Canola oil cooking spray
Fat-free sour cream or sugar-free or low-sugar fruit jams as garnish (optional)
Sugar-free syrup

In a mixing bowl combine pancake flour, milk, and canola oil. Using a wire whisk, mix ingredients until smooth. Add blueberries and walnuts and stir to combine all ingredients. Spray griddle with cooking spray and heat over medium heat. Drop a few droplets of water onto the heated griddle. If droplets bead, then griddle is hot enough. Pour about 1 tablespoon of batter per pancake onto griddle. Cook pancake until it begins to bubble up and edges turn brown, then flip over and continue cooking until the other side is golden brown. Remove cooked pancakes to a warmed platter or hold in a low-heat oven (175 degrees) while preparing other pancakes. Repeat this process until all the batter is gone. Serve with a dollop of fat-free sour cream or your favorite sugar-free syrup or low-sugar fruit jam if desired.

Approx. 85 calories per pancake
3g protein, 2g total fat, 0.5g saturated fat, 0 trans fat,
15g carbohydrates, 3mg cholesterol, 130mg sodium, 2g fiber

MULTIGRAIN APPLE AND NUT PANCAKES
(MAKES 6 PANCAKES)

¾ cup multigrain pancake flour
½ cup + 2 tablespoons skim milk
1 tablespoon canola oil
½ medium sweet apple, cored, peeled, and diced
⅛ cup chopped walnuts
Canola oil cooking spray
Fat-free sour cream or sugar-free or low-sugar fruit jams as garnish (optional)
Sugar-free syrup

In a mixing bowl combine pancake flour, milk, and canola oil. Using a wire whisk, mix ingredients until smooth. Add apple and walnuts and stir to combine all ingredients. Spray griddle with cooking spray and heat over medium heat. Drop a few droplets of water onto the heated griddle. If droplets bead, then griddle is hot enough. Pour about 1 tablespoon of batter per pancake onto griddle. Cook pancake until it begins to bubble up and edges turn brown, then flip over and continue cooking until the other side is golden brown. Remove cooked pancakes to a warmed platter or hold in a low-heat oven (175 degrees) while preparing other pancakes. Repeat this process until all the batter is gone. Serve with a dollop of fat-free sour cream or your favorite sugar-free syrup or low-sugar fruit jam if desired.

Approx. 87 calories per pancake
3g protein, 2g total fat, 0.5g saturated fat, 0 trans fat,
15g carbohydrates, 3mg cholesterol, 130mg sodium, 2g fiber

Main Dishes

SPICY SOLE
(MAKES 4 SERVINGS)

Spicy Pistachio Pesto (page 356)
8 (3-ounce) fillets of sole
1 cup water
1 cup dry white vermouth
1 tablespoon fresh lemon juice
Salt and freshly ground pepper to taste

Make pesto sauce and set aside. Season fillets with salt and pepper and roll up, securing with toothpicks. Set aside. Bring 1 cup water, vermouth, and lemon juice to a simmer; add rolled fillets, cover, and poach for about 7 minutes until flesh turns white and fish is cooked through. Remove rolled fillet from skillet with a slotted spoon. Serve plate immediately topped with Spicy Pistachio Pesto. Serve while hot.

Approx. 154 calories per 2 fillets
32g protein, 2g total fat, 0.6g saturated fat, 0 trans fat,
0 carbohydrates, 82mg cholesterol, 178mg sodium, 0 fiber

SPANISH PAELLA WITH SAFFRON RICE, SEAFOOD, AND CHICKEN

(makes 8 servings)

12 medium shrimp

7 hard-shelled clams

½ pound garlic-seasoned smoked pork sausage

2 pounds skinless, boneless chicken, cut into pieces

Dash of pepper

¾ teaspoon garlic salt

½ cup extra-virgin olive oil

¼ pound lean boneless pork, cut into ½-inch cubes

½ cup chopped onions

½ medium red bell pepper, seeded and sliced

½ medium yellow bell pepper, seeded and sliced

1 large tomato, peeled and finely chopped

2 cloves garlic, crushed

3 cups uncooked long-grain rice

½ teaspoon salt

¼ teaspoon ground saffron

6 cups water

1 cup frozen peas, thoroughly defrosted

Steam shrimp in a small amount of water until just pink, then set side. Scrub clams under running water, then steam in just enough water to cover them. When clams open, remove from water with a slotted spoon and set aside. Prick sausage with fork in several places, place in heavy skillet, and cover with cold water. Bring water to a boil and reduce heat to low. Simmer sausages, uncovered, for 15 minutes. Drain sausages well, slice into ¼-inch round pieces, and set aside. Rinse chicken, pat dry, and season with garlic salt and pepper. In a large skillet, heat ¼ cup olive oil, add chicken pieces, and fry until golden brown. Remove browned chicken from skillet and place on plate lined with paper towels. Add sausage pieces to skillet, quickly brown them, and then drain on plate lined with paper towels. Remove oil from skillet and dry skillet with paper towels. Add ¼ cup fresh olive oil and heat until hot. Add pork cubes and brown quickly. Add onions, red and yellow bell peppers, tomatoes, and garlic.

Cook vegetables and meat, stirring constantly, until tender. Set aside. In a large pot, add rice, salt, saffron, and 6 cups of water; bring to a boil and cover, stirring occasionally, until rice is soft. Transfer rice and remaining liquid, shrimp, clams, sausage, chicken and pork cubes, and vegetables to an oven-safe casserole dish. Sprinkle peas over mixture, place pan on bottom rack of a 400-degree oven, and bake for 25–30 minutes or until liquid is absorbed. Do not stir. When paella is cooked, remove from oven, cover with clean kitchen towel, and let stand for 5 minutes. Serve immediately. Note: oven should be preheated 30 minutes before paella is placed inside.

Approx. 523 calories per serving
38g protein, 13g total fat, 3g saturated fat, 0 trans fat,
61g carbohydrates, 117mg cholesterol, 819mg sodium, 3g fiber

SKEWERED MEDITERRANEAN GRILLED LAMB AND VEGETABLES
(MAKES 4 SERVINGS)

Juice from 2 lemons
⅓ cup extra-virgin olive oil
1 clove garlic, minced
1 tablespoon chopped mint
Salt and freshly ground pepper to taste
1½ pounds lamb sirloin, cut into 1½-inch cubes
8 large bay leaves
8 fresh mushroom caps
8 small cherry tomatoes
1 large green bell pepper, seeded and cut into 1½-inch strips
2 small zucchini, cut into 1-inch cubes
4 medium onions, quartered

Mix together lemon juice, olive oil, garlic, mint, and salt and pepper to taste, and pour over lamb cubes in a Ziploc bag. Place in refrigerator and marinate overnight or for at least 8 hours. On 8 flat-bladed oiled skewers alternate meat, bay leaves, and vegetables. Grill over hot coals for about 15 minutes, turning skewers several times.

This dish goes well with a chopped salad of onions, cucumbers, tomatoes, and parsley. Use lemon juice for dressing.

Approx. 296 calories per serving
38g protein, 8g total fat, 3g saturated fat, 0 trans fat,
15g carbohydrates, 103mg cholesterol, 141mg sodium, 3g fiber

BAKED STUFFED TROUT
(MAKES 4 SERVINGS)

4 (12-ounce) whole trout, scaled and gutted
3 tablespoons extra-virgin olive oil
1 large onion, finely chopped
4 cloves garlic, minced
⅔ cup plain bread crumbs
1 lemon, juiced and rind-grated
⅓ cup seedless dark raisins, chopped
½ cup pine nuts
2 tablespoons chopped fresh parsley
1 tablespoon chopped fresh dill
Salt and freshly ground pepper to taste
¼ cup egg substitute
Olive oil cooking spray
Lemon wedges for garnish

In a skillet heat 2 tablespoons of oil, add onion and garlic, and cook until soft, then remove from heat. In a large bowl, mix bread crumbs, grated lemon rind, raisins, pine nuts, parsley, dill, and salt and pepper; add garlic mixture and egg, and mix well together. Stuff each trout with mixture and place in a single layer on an oil-sprayed shallow baking pan. Make several diagonal slashes along the body of each fish and drizzle with lemon juice and remaining tablespoon of oil. Bake at 375 degrees for about 30–45 minutes or until fish flakes. Serve hot, garnished with lemon wedges.

Approx. 579 calories per serving
61g protein, 30g total fat, 5g saturated fat, 0 trans fat,
13g carbohydrates, 284mg cholesterol, 547mg sodium, 1g fiber

GREAT NORTHERN BEANS AND CHICKEN
(MAKES 6 SERVINGS)

2 (3-ounce) skinless, boneless chicken legs

2 (4-ounce) skinless, boneless chicken breasts

2 onions, chopped into large pieces

5 carrots, 1 sliced and others cut into large pieces

2 stalks celery, 1 sliced and other cut into large pieces

Olive oil cooking spray

2 cups low-sodium, fat-free chicken broth

4 cups canned Great Northern beans, drained and rinsed

2 tomatoes, peeled and chopped into large pieces

½ green bell pepper, chopped into large pieces

2 teaspoons fresh thyme

3 cloves fresh garlic, chopped

2 tablespoons chopped fresh parsley

Salt and freshly ground pepper to taste

Rinse chicken under water and pat dry. Place chicken, half of the onion, 1 sliced carrot, and 1 sliced celery stalk in a saucepan. Add water to cover chicken, and cook over medium heat until chicken is tender. Strain and set aside. Lightly spray bottom and sides of a large casserole dish with cooking spray, and add chicken, 2 cups of broth, and beans. Cut remaining carrots and celery into large pieces and add to casserole along with tomatoes, remaining onion, green pepper, thyme, garlic, parsley, and salt and pepper. Bake for 45 minutes, until mixture simmers. Serve while hot.

Approx. 352 calories per serving
34g protein, 7g total fat, 2g saturated fat, 0 trans fat,
39g carbohydrates, 82mg cholesterol, 267mg sodium, 2g fiber

BOUILLABAISSE
(MAKES 4 SERVINGS)

2 teaspoons extra-virgin olive oil

2 leeks, white and green parts, thinly sliced

3 cloves garlic, minced

2 cups freshly chopped tomatoes

¼ cup dry white wine

1 tablespoon tomato paste

1 tablespoon freshly chopped parsley

½ teaspoon dried thyme

2 bay leaves

⅓ teaspoon crushed saffron

⅛ teaspoon fennel seeds

10 ounces fresh firm cod, cut into 1½-inch chunks

2 (6-ounce) fresh lobster tails, quartered

16 littleneck clams, scrubbed

3 ounces orzo, cooked and drained

In a large saucepan over medium-high heat, combine oil, leek, and garlic; cook for about 3 minutes, stirring occasionally. Add tomatoes, 1½ cups of water, wine, tomato paste, parsley, thyme, bay leaves, saffron, and fennel seeds; stir to combine. Bring mixture to a boil, stirring occasionally. Add cod, lobster, and clams; return to boil. Reduce heat to low and simmer, covered, for 6–8 minutes. Fish and lobster should be cooked until done, and clams until they open. Remove bay leaf. Spoon cooked orzo into 4 soup bowls; ladle Bouillabaisse over orzo and serve.

Approx. 278 calories per serving
29g protein, 5g total fat, 1g saturated fat, 0 trans fat,
26g carbohydrates, 71mg cholesterol, 268mg sodium, 2g fiber

SPICY BROCCOLI RABE WITH PENNE PASTA
(MAKES 4 SERVINGS)

2 pounds fresh broccoli rabe, cleaned, trimmed, and cut into 1-inch pieces
1 pound whole wheat penne pasta
3 tablespoons extra-virgin olive oil
5 cloves garlic, thinly sliced
1 medium white onion, chopped
2 ounces anchovy fillets, drained
¼ teaspoon crushed red hot pepper
Salt and freshly ground pepper to taste
Freshly grated Romano cheese for garnish (optional)

In a large saucepan, bring water and salt to a boil. Add broccoli rabe and cook about 5 minutes, until stems are tender. With a slotted spoon, transfer broccoli to a colander to drain. Return broccoli water to a boil and add pasta. Cook until tender and drain, reserving ¼ cup of pasta water. Return pasta to a saucepan and keep warm. In a large skillet, heat oil, then add garlic and onion; sauté for about 2 minutes, until golden. Add anchovies and crushed red pepper, stirring for about 1 minute. Add broccoli rabe and cook another 5 minutes, until heated. To broccoli rabe mixture, add pasta and enough of reserved pasta liquid to lightly moisten; toss until well mixed. Add salt and pepper to taste. Garnish with Romano cheese. Serve warm.

Approx. 580 calories per serving
21g protein, 14g total fat, 2g saturated fat, 0 trans fat,
94g carbohydrates, 8mg cholesterol, 645mg sodium, 7g fiber

GRILLED CITRUS SALMON WITH GARLIC GREENS
(MAKES 4 SERVINGS)

¼ cup orange marmalade

2 tablespoons fresh lime juice

2 tablespoons fresh lemon juice

¼ cup low-sodium soy sauce

3 teaspoons grated orange rind

4 (3-ounce) salmon fillets

2 teaspoons extra-virgin olive oil

2 teaspoons minced garlic

2 (10-ounce) bags fresh spinach

Scant amount of olive oil to rub on fish

Salt and freshly ground pepper to taste

1 teaspoon fresh garlic, mashed to rub on fish

1 heaping tablespoon capers, drained

1 tablespoon balsamic vinegar

4 scallions, white and light green parts, thinly sliced (2–3 inch lengths)

Whisk together marmalade, lime and lemon juices, soy sauce, and orange rind; pour mixture over fillets and marinade for 30 minutes in refrigerator. Prepare grill or preheat broiler. Heat olive oil in a heavy skillet over medium-high heat; add garlic and spinach, one bag at a time, and sauté, stirring often, until spinach is wilted (about 2 minutes). Reduce heat to very low, to keep warm. Combine olive oil, salt and pepper, mashed garlic, and capers. Rub mixture into both sides of salmon steaks. Grill the fish or broil 3–4 inches from flame for 2–2 ½ minutes on each side. Set fish aside. Remove spinach from heat and toss with vinegar; divide equally on 4 plates. Add grilled salmon fillet to bed of spinach on each plate and garnish with onions. Serve.

Approx. 250 calories per serving
18g protein, 8g total fat, 1g saturated fat, 0 trans fat,
14g carbohydrates, 188mg cholesterol, 884mg sodium, 6g fiber

SICILIAN-STYLE LINGUINE WITH EGGPLANT AND ROASTED PEPPERS
(MAKES 6 SERVINGS)

2 large yellow bell peppers
1 small eggplant, peeled and cut into ½-inch cubes
2 tablespoons extra-virgin olive oil
2 tablespoons minced oregano
2 tablespoons capers
4 teaspoons minced garlic
1 (35-ounce) can peeled plum tomatoes
½ teaspoon red hot pepper flakes
Salt and fresh pepper to taste
1 pound linguine
1 cup shredded fresh basil leaves
¾ cup grated Romano cheese

Preheat broiler. Cut peppers in half and remove seeds. Cut each half into strips, and place on baking sheet, skin side up; broil until blackened. Set oven temperature to 400 degrees. Toss eggplant cubes with 1 tablespoon of oil, and place cubes in a single layer on a baking pan. Bake about 25 minutes, until very tender and browned, turning one time to bake evenly. Heat 1 tablespoon of oil in a large skillet over medium-high heat; add oregano, capers, and garlic, and sauté until garlic is lightly golden. Add eggplant, bell pepper, tomatoes and liquid, hot pepper flakes, and salt and pepper to taste. Cover, reduce heat, and simmer about 15 minutes, stirring occasionally. Cook pasta in boiling water, drain, and return it to the pot. Pour sauce over pasta, add basil, and gently toss. Sprinkle with cheese and serve.

Approx. 336 calories per serving
13g protein, 10g total fat, 3g saturated fat, 0 trans fat,
50g carbohydrates, 15mg cholesterol, 461mg sodium, 6g fiber

PENNE WITH ROSEMARY AND BALSAMIC VINEGAR
(MAKES 4 SERVINGS)

8 ounces penne pasta

2 teaspoons extra-virgin olive oil

2 cups zucchini, cut into ½-inch cubes

3–4 garlic cloves, minced

2 sprigs fresh rosemary, about 4–6 inches long

2 cups canned Italian peeled plum tomatoes, drained

1 tablespoon chopped fresh oregano

Salt and freshly ground pepper to taste

1 tablespoon balsamic vinegar

1 tablespoon + 1 teaspoon fresh grated Parmesan cheese

Bring water to a boil, add pasta, and cook pasta until *al dente*. Remove from heat, drain pasta, and return to pot, drizzling with scant amount of olive oil to keep pasta from sticking together. Set aside. In a large skillet, heat oil over medium-hot heat. Sauté zucchini, garlic, and rosemary (about 4–5 minutes). Add tomatoes, oregano, and salt and pepper to taste. Decrease heat to a simmer and cook for about 10–12 minutes. Add vinegar and mix well. Place cooked pasta into a bowl, pour sauce over pasta, and toss to mix. Sprinkle with Parmesan cheese and serve.

Approx. 231 calories per serving
9g protein, 3g total fat, 0.6g saturated fat, 0 trans fat,
42g carbohydrates, 1mg cholesterol, 235mg sodium, 3g fiber

CHICKEN AND EGGPLANT
(MAKES 8 SERVINGS)

2 medium eggplants, peeled and cut into 1½-inch cubes
½ cup extra-virgin olive oil
3 pounds skinless, boneless chicken
3 tablespoons extra-virgin olive oil
2 large onions, chopped
4 cloves garlic, chopped
1 teaspoon mixed spices

To make mixed spices combine:
2 teaspoons allspice
1 teaspoon ground cinnamon
1 teaspoon ground cloves
1 teaspoon cilantro
1 teaspoon ground cumin
¼ teaspoon freshly ground pepper

4 large tomatoes, peeled, seeded, and chopped
2 teaspoons Thick Pomegranate Molasses (page 354)
3 tablespoons fresh squeezed lemon juice
Salt and freshly ground pepper to taste
2 tablespoons finely chopped parsley

Salt eggplant pieces generously and let drain in a colander about 30 minutes (this rids eggplant of its bitter juices). After 30 minutes, rinse pieces under running cold water, gently squeeze pieces with hands to remove excess moisture, and pat dry with paper towels. In a large heavy skillet, heat olive oil over medium heat. Add half of the eggplant pieces and sauté, turning frequently until golden brown. With a slotted spoon, transfer pieces to paper towels to drain and soak up excess oil. Repeat procedure with remaining eggplant, adding more oil if necessary. Pour oil from skillet, allow to cool, and wipe clean. Rinse chicken pieces under cold water and pat dry with paper towels. Place chicken in skillet with 1 tablespoon of oil and sauté, turning to brown evenly on all sides. Transfer pieces to plate. Pour off all but 3 tablespoons of drippings from skillet. Add onions and sauté over moderate heat, until golden brown. Add garlic and mixed spices and sauté about 30 seconds while stirring. Add tomatoes, Thick Pomegranate Molasses, lemon juice, and salt and pepper to taste. Return chicken and any juices from plate to skillet, spooning tomato mixture around pieces. Bring to a boil and reduce to low. Cover and simmer about 45 minutes or until chicken is tender. Stir in sautéed eggplant and parsley, cover, and simmer an additional 10 minutes. Adjust seasonings to taste. Serve with a side dish of pasta (optional).

Approx. 376 calories per serving
37g protein, 24g total fat, 4g saturated fat, 0 trans fat,
2g carbohydrates, 120mg cholesterol, 133mg sodium, 0.4g fiber

SPICY WHOLE WHEAT CAPELLINI WITH GARLIC
(MAKES 4 SERVINGS)

8 ounces whole wheat capellini pasta
¼ cup extra-virgin olive oil
4 cloves garlic, chopped
1 teaspoon diced hot peppers
Salt and freshly ground pepper to taste
Grated Pecorino or Parmesan cheese (optional)

Bring water to a boil, add pasta, and cook pasta until *al dente*. Remove from heat, drain pasta, and return to pot, drizzling with scant amount of olive oil to keep pasta from sticking together. Set aside. In a heavy skillet over medium heat, add olive oil, then sauté garlic and hot pepper until tender (about 1–2 minutes). Add to pasta and toss. Add salt and pepper to taste, and sprinkle with grated cheese if desired.

Approx. 299 calories per serving
8g protein, 16g total fat, 2g saturated fat, 0 trans fat,
35g carbohydrates, 4mg cholesterol, 0 sodium, 7g fiber

BROILED RED SNAPPER WITH GARLIC
(MAKES 4 SERVINGS)

1 whole red snapper (about 2–2 ½ pounds), scaled and gutted
3 tablespoons lemon juice
1 cup dry white wine
1 chili pepper, chopped
3 cloves garlic, finely chopped
2 tablespoons extra-virgin olive oil
Salt and freshly ground pepper to taste
Olive oil cooking spray
2 tablespoons chopped fresh oregano
2 tablespoons chopped fresh parsley
Lemon wedges

Marinate cleaned fish for 1 hour in the refrigerator in a shallow pan with 1 tablespoon lemon juice, wine, chili pepper, and 1 clove chopped garlic. Preheat broiler. Whisk together the remaining lemon juice, oil, and salt and pepper. Rub inside and outside of fish with mixture. Place fish on an oil-sprayed broiler pan and sprinkle with oregano. Broil fish for about 10 minutes, basting often with oil mixture and turning once, until golden brown. Meanwhile, mix together remaining 2 cloves of chopped garlic and parsley. Sprinkle the parsley mixture on top of cooked fish and serve hot, garnished with lemon wedges.

Approx. 185 calories per serving
25g protein, 11g total fat, 2g saturated fat, 0 trans fat,
0 carbohydrates, 46mg cholesterol, 81mg sodium, 0 fiber

PASTA WITH PINE NUTS AND SCALLOPS
(MAKES 4 SERVINGS)

8 ounces tagliatelle or fettuccine
4 tablespoons extra-virgin olive oil
3 cloves garlic, finely chopped
1 leek, white part only, thinly sliced
10 pitted black olives, halved
¼ cup pine nuts
12 large sea scallops, halved
Salt and freshly ground pepper to taste
2 tablespoons chopped fresh basil
Parmesan cheese, finely grated, for garnish (optional)

Bring water to a boil, add pasta, and cook pasta until *al dente*. Remove from heat, drain pasta, and return to pot, drizzling with scant amount of olive oil to keep pasta from sticking together. Set aside. While pasta is cooking, heat olive oil in a skillet, add garlic and leek, and cook until soft but not brown. Add olives and pine nuts, and sauté until pine nuts are lightly browned. Add scallops, and cook until scallops are opaque. Add salt and pepper to taste. Add scallops and pan juices to pasta and toss. Sprinkle with basil and garnish with cheese if desired.

Approx. 409 calories per serving
17g protein, 23g total fat, 3g saturated fat, 0 trans fat,
41g carbohydrates, 45mg cholesterol, 139mg sodium, 1g fiber

SPICY SHRIMP WITH ANGEL HAIR PASTA
(MAKES 4 SERVINGS)

8 ounces angel hair pasta
1½ pounds medium shrimp, peeled and deveined
1 teaspoon low-calorie baking sweetener
¼ teaspoon salt
1 tablespoon chili powder
½ teaspoon ground cumin
½ teaspoon ground coriander
½ teaspoon dried oregano
1 tablespoon + 1 teaspoon extra-virgin olive oil
Lime wedges for garnish

Bring water to a boil, add pasta, and cook pasta until *al dente*. Remove from heat, drain pasta, and return to pot, drizzling with scant amount of olive oil to keep pasta from sticking together. Set aside. Sprinkle shrimp with sweetener and salt. Combine chili powder, cumin, coriander, and oregano, then lightly coat shrimp with spice mixture. Heat 1 tablespoon of olive oil in a large non-stick skillet over medium-high heat. Add half of the shrimp and sauté about 4 minutes, or until cooked. Remove cooked shrimp from pan and repeat procedure with 1 teaspoon olive oil and remaining shrimp. Divide cooked pasta into 4 servings, top with shrimp and pan sauce, and garnish with lime wedges. Serve immediately.

Approx. 320 calories per serving
28g protein, 5g total fat, 0.6g saturated fat, 0 trans fat,
28g carbohydrates, 161mg cholesterol, 759mg sodium, 5g fiber

FRUIT-GLAZED SALMON WITH COUSCOUS
(MAKES 4 SERVINGS)

¾ pound couscous

2 cups low-sodium, fat-free chicken broth, heated

½ cup apricot jam

3 tablespoons thinly sliced scallion

2 tablespoons prepared horseradish

1 tablespoon white wine vinegar

½ teaspoon salt (divided)

4 (6-ounce) salmon fillets, 1-inch thick, skinned

¼ teaspoon freshly ground pepper

2 teaspoons extra-virgin olive oil

Oil an oven-safe dish and place couscous in dish. Pour in chicken broth and let sit for 10 minutes until couscous is tender and liquid is absorbed. Cover dish and keep warm in a low-temperature oven until ready to serve. Meanwhile, combine apricot jam, scallions, horseradish, vinegar, and ¼ teaspoon of salt, and stir well with a whisk. Sprinkle salmon fillets with ¼ teaspoon of salt and pepper. Heat olive oil in a large non-stick skillet over medium-high heat. Add salmon and cook for 3 minutes. Turn salmon and brush with half of apricot mixture. Wrap skillet handle with foil and bake salmon in skillet at 350 degrees for 5 minutes or until fish flakes. Remove from oven and brush salmon with remaining apricot mixture. Serve each fillet with couscous.

Approx. 396 calories per salmon fillet only
34g protein, 13g total fat, 2g saturated fat, 0 trans fat,
25g carbohydrates, 94mg cholesterol, 344mg sodium, 0 fiber

Approx. 198 calories per serving couscous only
7g protein, 0 total fat, 0 saturated fat, 0 trans fat,
40g carbohydrates, 0 cholesterol, 184mg sodium, 2g fiber

PASTA PRIMAVERA WITH SHRIMP
(MAKES 4 SERVINGS)

1 pound whole wheat penne pasta
½ cup low-sodium, fat-free chicken broth
1 tablespoon + 1 teaspoon extra-virgin olive oil
2 dozen medium shrimp, cleaned, peeled, and deveined
1½ cups broccoli florets
1 medium red bell pepper, thinly sliced
1 cup halved button mushrooms
1 cup frozen peas
½ cup sliced scallions
4 cloves fresh garlic, minced
1 ounce (2 tablespoons) dry white wine
2 tablespoons freshly grated Parmesan cheese

Bring water to a boil, add pasta, and cook pasta until *al dente*. Remove from heat, drain pasta, and return to pot, drizzling with scant amount of olive oil to keep pasta from sticking together. Set aside. In a large nonstick skillet, heat ¼ cup broth, 2 teaspoons of olive oil, and shrimp; cook until shrimp are pink. With a slotted spoon remove shrimp and set aside. To skillet add remaining ¼ cup of broth, broccoli, pepper, mushrooms, peas, scallions, and garlic. Cook, stirring frequently, for 4–5 minutes, until vegetables are tender and liquid is mostly absorbed. Stir in wine and simmer roughly 1 minute longer and add shrimp to vegetable mixture. Place penne pasta in a large serving bowl and toss with remaining olive oil. Add vegetable mixture; toss to mix well. Sprinkle with Parmesan cheese.

Approx. 526 calories per serving
24g protein, 8g total fat, 1g saturated fat, 0 trans fat,
78g carbohydrates, 34mg cholesterol, 218mg sodium, 12g fiber

TURKISH MUSSEL STEW
(MAKES 6–8 SERVINGS)

1 cup dry white wine
1 cup water
6 dozen mussels, scrubbed and debearded (discard any open mussels)
1 medium onion, peeled and sliced
1 leek, white part only, sliced
6 cloves garlic, coarsely chopped
¼ cup extra-virgin olive oil
4 large tomatoes, peeled and diced
2 large white potatoes, peeled, sliced about ¼-inch thick
2 medium carrots, cleaned and chunked
Pinch of saffron
2 bay leaves
Salt and freshly ground pepper to taste
¼ cup finely chopped flat leaf parsley

In a large heavy saucepan combine wine, water, and mussels. Cover pan and steam mussels until they open (roughly about 7–10 minutes). Remove mussels from liquid and discard any that have not opened. Set mussel liquid aside. Remove mussels from shells and add a small amount of liquid to keep them moist. Strain remaining mussel liquid through cheesecloth and set aside. In a clean saucepan, gently sauté onion, leek, and garlic until tender, then add tomatoes and cook for another 1–2 minutes. Add potato slices, carrots, saffron, bay leaves, and strained mussel liquid; cover pan and cook over medium-low heat until vegetables are tender (about 30 minutes). Add mussels to mixture and continue cooking until all is heated thoroughly; add salt and pepper to taste. Remove from heat and stir in parsley. Serve while hot.

Approx. 236 calories per serving
14g protein, 9g total fat, 1g saturated fat, 0 trans fat,
20g carbohydrates, 28mg cholesterol, 297mg sodium, 1g fiber

PESTO STUFFED SHELLS
(MAKES 4 SERVINGS)

3 ounces (about 12) jumbo pasta shells
1 tablespoon extra-virgin olive oil
2 cloves garlic, finely minced
1 cup thinly sliced button mushrooms
¼ teaspoon thyme
1 cup red bell pepper, diced
½ cup yellow summer squash, diced
1 can (15 ounces) chickpeas, rinsed and drained
½ cup sliced leek, white and green parts
1 cup part-skim ricotta cheese
Basil Pesto Sauce (page 357), or market-fresh pesto sauce
Grated Parmesan cheese to taste, for garnish

Bring water to a boil, add pasta, and cook pasta until *al dente*. Remove from heat, drain pasta, and return to pot, drizzling with scant amount of olive oil to keep pasta from sticking together. Set aside. Heat olive oil in a large skillet over medium-high heat. Add garlic, mushrooms, and thyme, and sauté about 6 minutes. Add bell pepper and squash, then cook mixture until vegetables are crispy tender. Remove from heat; stir in chickpeas and leek. Add ricotta cheese and ⅓ cup of pesto sauce, then gently stir mixture. Spoon mixture evenly into cooked shells and garnish with grated Parmesan cheese if desired.

Approx. 404 calories per serving
14g protein, 24g total fat, 6g saturated fat, 0 trans fat,
39g carbohydrates, 23mg cholesterol, 356mg sodium, 5g fiber

STEAMED SEA BASS
(MAKES 6 SERVINGS)

2 pounds sea bass (or grouper), 1-inch-thick whole fillets if possible
2½ tablespoons extra-virgin olive oil
8 thin slices red onion
2 cloves garlic, thinly sliced
10 medium dill sprigs
8 lemon slices, ½-inch thick
1 tablespoon capers, rinsed and drained
Freshly ground pepper to taste
2 tablespoons dry white wine
Sea salt to taste
Parchment paper

Cut parchment paper twice the size of fish and place on a baking sheet. Center fish on paper and drizzle with olive oil. Scatter onion slices, garlic, dill sprigs, and lemon slices on top of fish. Add capers and sprinkle with freshly ground pepper and a splash of wine. Wrap parchment paper around fish, folding top and tucking ends under fish to form a seal so steam cannot escape while baking. Bake in a 400-degree oven for 30 minutes. Check after 20 minutes for doneness; fish should be opaque in the center. If not, rewrap tightly and continue baking for an additional 10 minutes. To serve, place fish, still wrapped in parchment, on a platter. Open parchment when ready to serve; sprinkle on salt and serve immediately.

This dish goes well with rice, steamed vegetables, and/or couscous.

Approx. 205 calories per serving
28g protein, 7g total fat, 0.7g saturated fat, 0 trans fat,
4g carbohydrates, 62mg cholesterol, 103mg sodium, 0 fiber

TAHINI BAKED FLOUNDER
(MAKES 4 SERVINGS)

4 (3-ounce) fillets of flounder
2 tablespoons low-sodium soy sauce
2 tablespoons tahini paste
¼ cup fresh lemon juice
2 tablespoons extra-virgin olive oil
Freshly ground pepper to taste
2 oranges, peeled and sliced

Place fillets in a baking pan. Whisk together soy sauce, tahini paste, lemon juice, oil, and pepper. Pour mixture over fish and top fish with orange slices; cover and bake at 400 degrees for about 20–25 minutes or until fish flakes, then serve hot.

This dish goes well with steamed vegetables and rice.

Approx. 312 calories per serving
21g protein, 22g total fat, 3.2g saturated fat, 0 trans fat,
7.8g carbohydrates, 42mg cholesterol, 182mg sodium, 2g fiber

SPICY CHICKEN WITH COUSCOUS
(MAKES 4 SERVINGS)

¼ teaspoon ground cumin
¼ teaspoon ground turmeric
1 teaspoon ground cayenne
1 teaspoon extra-virgin olive oil
1 pound skinless, boneless chicken breasts, cut into 1-inch strips
5 cloves garlic, finely minced
1 (16-ounce) can low-sodium, fat-free chicken broth
1 cup fresh peas
1 large white onion, diced
1 medium red bell pepper, diced
Salt and freshly ground pepper to taste
1 cup uncooked couscous
¼ cup chopped fresh cilantro, for garnish

Combine cumin, turmeric, and cayenne, and sprinkle evenly over chicken strips, then set aside. In a non-stick skillet, add oil and heat over medium-high heat until hot. Add chicken and garlic, and cook about 3 minutes until chicken is lightly browned. Add broth, peas, onion, and red pepper to skillet; bring to boil, reduce heat, and simmer about 2–3 minutes, until chicken is cooked through. Stir in couscous, cover, and remove from heat. Let stand until liquid is absorbed. Garnish with cilantro.

Approx. 340 calories per serving
34g protein, 4g total fat, 0.6g saturated fat, 0 trans fat,
38g carbohydrates, 66mg cholesterol, 746mg sodium, 3g fiber

CITRUS SCALLOPS AND SHRIMP

(MAKES 4 SERVING)

3 cloves garlic, finely minced
2½ tablespoons extra-virgin olive oil
1½ pounds fresh arugula
½ pound large sea scallops, cut in halves
12 large shrimp, peeled and deveined
4 ounces fresh orange juice
Juice from ½ pink grapefruit
Juice from 1 lime
Juice from 1 lemon
1 teaspoon honey
½ teaspoon finely shredded orange zest
½ teaspoon finely shredded lime zest
¼ tablespoon extra-virgin olive oil
Salt and freshly ground pepper to taste
2 scallions, sliced thin

In a large skillet over medium-high heat, sauté garlic in 1 tablespoon of olive oil for 1 minute; do not brown. Add arugula, cover, and cook 1 minute, until greens are wilted. In a separate skillet, over medium-high heat, heat remaining oil. Add scallops and shrimp, and cook until scallops are opaque and shrimp pink, gently turning to keep from burning. Transfer scallops and shrimp to a heated plate, cover to keep warm, and set aside. Reserve skillet with seafood drippings, and set aside. Combine orange juice, grapefruit juice, lime juice, lemon juice, honey, and orange and lime zest. Pour juice mixture into reserved seafood skillet, and return skillet to medium heat. Stir the bottom and sides of pan to loosen any browned bits, incorporating them into juices. Bring to a boil, and cook until liquid is reduced to half amount. Add salt and pepper to taste, cook for a few seconds, and remove from heat. Drain wilted arugula and divide between 4 plates, mounding in center. Divide scallops and shrimp into four portions, and arrange on top of arugula. Pour juice glaze over seafood and garnish with sliced scallions.

Approx. 309 calories per serving
34g protein, 11g total fat, 1g saturated fat, 0 trans fat,
26g carbohydrates, 45mg cholesterol, 276mg sodium, 2g fiber

ITALIAN POACHED SCALLOPS
(MAKES 4 SERVINGS)

1 cup fresh orange juice
1 pound fresh sea scallops
2 teaspoons grated orange peel
1 small ripe plum tomato, chopped
1 teaspoon chopped fresh marjoram
2 tablespoons low-fat sour cream
Salt to taste
Freshly ground pepper

In a large nonstick skillet over medium heat, bring orange juice to a boil. Reduce heat, and add scallops and orange peels. Cover and simmer 5 minutes or until scallops are opaque and tender. Remove scallops from heat and transfer to a plate; cover to keep warm. Add tomatoes and marjoram to orange juice sauce and simmer for roughly 2 minutes until liquid reduces to half of original amount. Stir in sour cream, and cook until sauce thickens. Add salt and pepper to taste. Return scallops to skillet, mix with sauce, and heat through. Serve immediately with risotto and/or vegetables.

Approx. 148 calories per serving
16g protein, 2g total fat, 0.5g saturated fat, 0 trans fat,
11g carbohydrates, 34mg cholesterol, 380mg sodium, 1g fiber

GRILLED GROUPER
(MAKES 4 SERVINGS)

½ cup ripe pitted Kalamata olives
¼ cup plain bread crumbs
1 tablespoon capers, rinsed and drained
1 teaspoon extra-virgin olive oil
1 teaspoon lemon juice
1 clove garlic
4 (4-ounce) grouper fillets
4–8 lime wedges for garnish

Heat grill to high heat; place oil-rubbed fish-grilling pan on grill rack to heat. In a food processor, process olives, bread crumbs, capers, olive oil, lemon juice, and garlic until smooth. Brush each side of fillets with olive oil mixture and place fillet on hot grill pan. Grill fillets, uncovered, for 5 minutes. Before turning fillets over, brush with olive oil mixture, then turn and grill for additional 5 minutes or until fillets flake easily. Remove fillets from grill, place on platter, and serve immediately, garnished with lime wedges.

This dish goes well with seasoned rice or couscous.

Approx. 159 calories per serving
24g protein, 4g total fat, <0.4g saturated fat, 0 trans fat,
4g carbohydrates, 45mg cholesterol, 388mg sodium, 0 fiber

SPICY STUFFED TILAPIA
(MAKES 4 SERVINGS)

4 (4-ounce) tilapia fillets
2 cups prepared crab meat stuffing mix (¼ cup per fillet)
5 ounces fresh spinach leaves, rinsed and drained
1 tablespoon extra-virgin olive oil
½ teaspoon fresh crushed garlic
Sea salt and freshly ground pepper to taste
¼ cup dry-roasted pistachios, crushed
Red hot pepper sauce to drizzle

Rinse tilapia fillets under cold water and pat dry. Divide stuffing mix between 4 fillets, placing mix on the center of each fillet. Fold fillets over and secure with wooden skewers. Spread spinach on a baking sheet. Place stuffed fillets on bed of spinach. Drizzle fillets with olive oil, scatter with garlic, and season with sea salt and freshly ground pepper to taste. Scatter pistachios evenly over fillets and drizzle red hot pepper sauce over top. Bake at 350 degrees for 20–30 minutes or until fish flakes easily. Serve immediately.

Approx. 243 calories per serving
18g protein, 11g total fat, 5g saturated fat, 0 trans fat,
3.5g carbohydrates, 104mg cholesterol, 558mg sodium, 1g fiber

BAKED TILAPIA
(MAKES 2 SERVINGS)

4 (4-ounce) tilapia fillets
2 tablespoons extra-virgin olive oil
3 cloves garlic, minced
2 scallions, white and green parts, chopped
½ cup fresh chopped parsley
Salt and freshly ground pepper to taste
Fresh spinach leaves and 6 grape tomatoes, halved, for garnish
Juice from 2 lemons
1 lemon, quartered

Rinse fillets under cold water and pat dry. Place fillets in a baking dish. In mixing bowl combine oil, garlic, scallions, and parsley; pour over fish, cover, and refrigerate for 30 minutes. Sprinkle with salt and pepper and bake at 350 degrees for 15 minutes or until fish flakes easily. Divide cleaned spinach on 2 plates. Remove fish from oven, and place 2 fillets on top of spinach on each plate. Garnish each plate with tomato halves. Squeeze juice from 2 lemons over fillets, garnish with lemon wedge, and serve.

Approx. 138 calories per serving (two fillets per serving)
15g protein, 8g total fat, 1g saturated fat, 0 trans fat,
3g carbohydrates, 43mg cholesterol, 46mg sodium, 0 fiber

SPICY RIGATONI WITH MUSSELS
(MAKES 6 SERVINGS)

1 pound rigatoni pasta
½ cup dry white wine
2 pounds mussels, scrubbed and debearded (discard any open mussels)
2 tablespoons extra-virgin olive oil
2 cloves garlic, minced
1½ cups cherry tomatoes, halved
1 teaspoon hot red peppers, diced (optional)
Salt and freshly ground pepper to taste
10–12 arugula leaves, chopped

Bring water to a boil, add pasta, and cook pasta until *al dente*. Remove from heat, drain pasta, and return to pot, drizzling with scant amount of olive oil to keep pasta from sticking together. Set aside. In another pot over high heat, add wine and mussels. Cook until mussels open. Discard any that do not open. Remove cooked mussels from liquid. Set aside. Sieve mussel liquid, reserve liquid only. Shell mussels except for 12 mussels (to be used for garnish). In large skillet heat oil, add garlic, and sauté. Add tomatoes and hot pepper, sauté for a few minutes. Add shelled mussels and 3–4 teaspoons of mussel liquid, season mixture with salt to taste. Place pasta in a large pasta server, fluff noodles with a fork, and toss with garlic mussel mixture. Scatter chopped arugula leaves over top, garnish with unshelled mussels, and serve.

Approx. 454 calories per serving
31g protein, 10g total fat, 1g saturated fat, 0 trans fat,
54g carbohydrates, 44mg cholesterol, 463mg sodium, 8g fiber

LINGUINE AND MIXED SEAFOOD
(MAKES 4–6 SERVINGS)

8 ounces natural clam juice
2 cups good dry wine (not cooking wine)
¼ pound baby octopus, cleaned
¼ pound shrimp, peeled and deveined
¼ pound calamari, cleaned, cut into ¼-inch rings
20 mussels, scrubbed and debearded (discard any open mussels)
¼ pound bay scallops
3 tablespoons extra-virgin olive oil
3–4 cloves garlic, minced
¼ teaspoon freshly chopped hot peppers
8 small ripe plum tomatoes, chopped into small chunks
Pinch of low-calorie baking sweetener
½ tablespoon chopped fresh parsley
½ tablespoon chopped fresh oregano
Salt and freshly ground pepper to taste
½ pound linguine
10–12 arugula leaves, chopped
10 pitted Kalamata black olives, halved

In a large deep skillet, add clam juice, wine, octopus, shrimp, calamari, mussels, and scallops. Bring to boil, cover, and reduce heat to simmer, stirring occasionally, until calamari and squid are almost tender.
Remove mussels and shell all but 9–12; set these aside for garnish and
return shelled mussels to seafood skillet to keep warm. In a separate skillet, over medium heat, add oil and garlic, and sauté until golden brown.
Add hot peppers to garlic mixture, reduce heat to simmer, and cook for
1–2 additional minutes. Add tomatoes, sweetener, parsley, oregano, and
salt and pepper to taste, and simmer another 3–4 minutes. Cover to keep
warm, and set aside. Bring water to a boil, add pasta, and cook pasta until
al dente. Remove from heat, drain pasta, and return to pot, drizzling with
scant amount of olive oil to keep pasta from sticking together. Set aside.
With a slotted spoon remove seafood from skillet and strain remaining
liquid through sieve or cheesecloth. Return seafood and 1 cup of strained
liquid to skillet; add pasta and tomato mixture, and toss all ingredients.

Spoon entire linguini and seafood dish into a large pasta bowl, garnish with chopped arugula, black olives, and remaining unshelled mussels, and serve.

Approx. 375 calories per serving
21g protein, 8g total fat, 1g saturated fat, 0 trans fat,
34g carbohydrates, 98mg cholesterol, 235mg sodium, 2g fiber

LAMB AND BLACK OLIVES
(MAKES 4–6 SERVINGS)

2 tablespoons extra-virgin olive oil
3 cloves garlic, crushed
1–2 sprigs fresh parsley
2 pounds ground lean lamb
2 tomatoes, peeled and chopped
½ teaspoon dried rosemary
12 pitted black olives, halved
1 cup dry white wine

Heat olive oil in a large skillet; add garlic and parsley, and sauté until golden brown. Add lamb, continuing to cook, and stir often until lamb is browned. Add tomatoes, rosemary, olives, and wine. Stir, cover, and cook 3–5 minutes or until lamb is cooked through and most of liquid has evaporated. Serve with rice.

Approx. 461 calories per serving
62g protein, 21g total fat, 6g saturated fat, 0 trans fat,
203mg cholesterol, 262mg sodium, 0.5g fiber

RIGATONI WITH GROUND LAMB
(MAKES 6–8 SERVINGS)

1 pound ground lean lamb
1 whole onion, minced
½ teaspoon dried hot red pepper flakes
1½ cups frozen peas
2 tablespoons Spicy Garlicky Pesto Sauce (page 354)
Salt and freshly ground pepper to taste
1 pound whole grain rigatoni pasta
2–3 tablespoons fresh chopped mint

In a heavy-bottomed saucepan cook lamb, onions, and red pepper flakes for about 8 minutes, until lamb is cooked, stirring occasionally to break up meat. Add frozen peas and cook for another 2–4 minutes. Add Spicy Garlicky Pesto Sauce, salt and pepper to taste, mix well, and set aside; keep warm. Cook rigatoni in boiling water until *al dente*, drain pasta, and toss with lamb pesto sauce. Garnish with fresh chopped mint.

Approx. 340 calories per serving
20g protein, 7.5g total fat, 1.5g saturated fat, 0 trans fat,
45g carbohydrates, 38mg cholesterol, 64mg sodium, 1g fiber

BOW TIE PASTA WITH EGGPLANT AND BLACK OLIVES
(MAKES 6–8 SERVINGS)

1 pound bow tie pasta
1 small eggplant, peeled and cut into 1–2-inch strips
Salt to taste
3 tablespoons extra-virgin olive oil
1 medium onion, chopped
Pinch of crushed red pepper flakes
6 cloves garlic, minced
½ teaspoon dried oregano
4 tablespoons freshly chopped basil
12 pitted black olives, Nicoise or Kalamata, chopped
Freshly ground pepper to taste
4 ounces crumbled feta cheese
Chopped parsley

Bring water to a boil, add pasta, and cook pasta until *al dente*. Remove from heat, drain pasta, and return to pot, drizzling with scant amount of olive oil to keep pasta from sticking together. Set aside. Salt eggplant strips and microwave to reduce water content in eggplant. Squeeze each piece between paper towels to remove excess water. Heat oil over medium heat and sauté onions and red pepper flakes for 1–2 minutes. Add eggplant, garlic, and oregano and sauté until eggplant is lightly browned. Add basil, olives, and salt and pepper to taste. Transfer pasta to a serving bowl and toss with eggplant mixture. Serve garnished with feta cheese and chopped parsley.

Approx. 308 calories per serving
10g protein, 10g total fat, 3g saturated fat, 0 trans fat,
52g carbohydrates, 13mg cholesterol, 256mg sodium, 2g fiber

PASTA WITH RED CLAM SAUCE
(MAKES 6–8 SERVINGS)

1 pound whole grain angel hair pasta
1 cup dry white wine
4 ounces bottled clam juice
3 cloves fresh garlic, finely chopped
¼ teaspoon dried basil
48 small hard-shell clams, cleaned (discard any open clams)
2 tablespoons extra-virgin olive oil
½ white onion, chopped
1 pound whole tomatoes, peeled, seeded, and chopped
¼ teaspoon dried oregano
Salt and freshly ground pepper to taste
1 teaspoon chopped parsley

Bring water to a boil, add pasta, and cook pasta until *al dente*. Remove from heat, drain pasta, and return to pot, drizzling with scant amount of olive oil to keep pasta from sticking together. Set aside. In a large skillet heat wine and clam juice, add 1 clove chopped garlic, basil, and clams in their shells, cover, and steam until shells open. Remove clams from liquid and discard any unopened clams. Strain liquid through strainer to remove grit, and set liquid aside. Reserve 16 clams in their shells for garnish, then remove remaining clams from shells and return them to strained liquid. In a separate skillet, heat oil, add onion and remaining garlic, and sauté until golden. Add tomatoes, oregano, and salt and pepper to garlic mixture and cook for 8 minutes. Add shelled clams with strained liquid to tomato mixture and heat through for another 2–3 minutes, stirring to blend tastes. Pour clam sauce over pasta, toss, and garnish with reserved unshelled clams and parsley.

Approx. 284 calories per serving
23g protein, 6g total fat, 0.6g saturated fat, 0 trans fat,
47g carbohydrates, 46mg cholesterol, 82mg sodium, 6g fiber

PASTA WITH CLAMS, WINE, AND RED HOT PEPPERS
(MAKES 6–8 SERVINGS)

1 pound whole grain spaghetti
1 cup dry white wine
4 ounces bottled clam juice
48 small hard-shell clams, cleaned (discard any open clams)
2 tablespoons extra-virgin olive oil
3 cloves fresh garlic, finely chopped
1 small hot chili pepper, minced
4 tablespoons finely chopped fresh parsley
Salt and freshly ground pepper to taste

Bring water to a boil, add pasta, and cook pasta until *al dente*. Remove from heat, drain pasta, and return to pot, drizzling with scant amount of olive oil to keep pasta from sticking together. Set aside. In a large skillet, heat wine and clam juice, add clams in their shells, cover, and steam until shells open. Remove clams from liquid and discard any unopened clams. Strain liquid through strainer to remove grit and set aside. Reserve 16 clams in their shells for garnish; remove remaining clams from shells and return them to strained liquid. Set aside reserved unshelled clams. In a large skillet heat oil, garlic, chilies, and parsley, bring to a sizzle, and add shelled clams with strained juice, and salt and pepper to taste; stir and heat through. Pour sauce over pasta, toss, and garnish with reserved unshelled clams.

Approx. 308 calories per serving
28g protein, 7g total fat, 0.7g saturated fat, 0 trans fat,
49g carbohydrates, 51mg cholesterol, 86mg sodium, 7g fiber

WHOLE WHEAT SPAGHETTI WITH ANCHOVY AND GARLIC SAUCE

(MAKES 6–8 SERVINGS)

1 pound whole wheat spaghetti
6 tablespoons extra-virgin olive oil + oil from anchovies
6 large cloves fresh garlic, pressed
2-ounce tin of anchovy fillets packed in oil, drained and chopped
Red hot pepper flakes to taste
6–8 pitted black olives, chopped
2 tablespoons finely chopped parsley
Freshly ground pepper to taste
Romano cheese, finely grated (optional)

Bring water to a boil, add pasta, and cook pasta until *al dente*. Remove from heat, drain pasta, and return to pot, drizzling with scant amount of olive oil to keep pasta from sticking together. Set aside. Combine both oils and garlic in a skillet over medium heat and cook about 1–2 minutes. Add anchovies, breaking into small pieces and stirring to blend well with other ingredients. Cook about 30 seconds and remove from heat. Fold in hot pepper flakes, chopped black olives, and parsley. Place pasta in a large pasta serving bowl, add anchovy sauce, and toss to mix. Add pepper to taste, sprinkle with a small amount of grated Romano cheese if desired, and serve.

Approx. 347 calories per serving
14g protein, 16g total fat, 1g saturated fat, 0 trans fat,
39g carbohydrates, 11mg cholesterol, 244mg sodium, 6g fiber

FETTUCCINE WITH SUNDRIED TOMATOES AND GOAT CHEESE
(MAKES 6–8 SERVINGS)

4 tablespoons chopped sundried tomatoes (in olive oil)
1 cup sliced scallions
4 garlic cloves, minced
1 medium red bell pepper, thinly sliced
½ cup dry vermouth
¼ cup chopped fresh basil
10 pitted Kalamata olives
1 tablespoon capers, rinsed and drained
2 teaspoons dried oregano
1 pound whole wheat fettuccine, cooked and drained
6 ounces crumbled low-fat goat cheese

Drain oil from tomatoes and reserve oil; set tomatoes aside. In a large skillet, heat oil from tomatoes over medium heat. Add scallions and garlic to oil and sauté until soft. Add red peppers and ¼ cup of vermouth to garlic mixture. Cook peppers until crispy tender or until vermouth is almost evaporated. Reduce heat to simmer, and add tomatoes, remaining ¼ cup of vermouth, basil, olives, capers, and oregano. Simmer, stirring often to incorporate flavors (about 5–8 minutes), then reduce to very low heat to keep warm. Cook pasta to desired consistency (*al dente* would be best), and drain. Place pasta in a large bowl and toss with goat cheese until well blended. Add tomato mixture and toss again until well mixed. Serve.

Approx. 269 calories per serving
12g protein, 6g total fat, 2g saturated fat, 0 trans fat,
44g carbohydrates, 4mg cholesterol, 323mg sodium, 7g fiber

FLORENTINE ROASTED PORK
(MAKES 6–8 SERVINGS)

4 pounds lean loin pork
4 cloves garlic, sliced thin
½ teaspoon dried rosemary
4 cloves garlic, whole
5–6 tablespoons water
6–8 tablespoons hearty red wine (do not use a cooking wine)
Salt and freshly ground pepper to taste

If the skin of the loin has not already been scored, cut lines into skin about ⅛ inch apart. Cut through the flesh to the bone on one side and insert the garlic slices and rosemary. Press the cloves into the scored skin of the loin and place loin into a roasting pan in a 350-degree oven with water and wine. Sprinkle loin generously with salt and pepper and roast for 2–2 ½ hours or until meat is very tender but still moist, basting occasionally. Serve with a variety of your favorite vegetables.

Approx. 352 calories per serving
47g protein, 17g total fat, 5.6g saturated fat, 0 trans fat,
0 carbohydrates, 136mg cholesterol, 144mg sodium, 0 fiber

CHICKEN WITH POMEGRANATE SAUCE
(MAKES 6–8 SERVINGS)

4 pounds skinless, boneless chicken breast, cut into small pieces
2 teaspoons paprika
Salt and freshly ground pepper to taste
¼ cup extra-virgin olive oil
4 cloves fresh garlic, minced
2 medium yellow onions, chopped
¼ cup chopped fresh parsley
1 small hot banana pepper, finely chopped
3 tablespoons Thick Pomegranate Molasses (page 354)
3–4 cups canned chunky tomatoes, with liquid

Wash chicken, remove fat, and cut into small pieces. Sprinkle with paprika and salt and pepper. Heat oil in a saucepan, add chicken pieces, and stir-fry for about 2–3 minutes. Add garlic and stir-fry for another 2–3 minutes. Add onion, parsley, hot pepper, Thick Pomegranate Molasses, and tomatoes with liquid; cover and bring to boil. Cook over medium-low heat for about 30 minutes until chicken is tender. Serve with rice.

Approx. 364 calories per serving
50g protein, 14g total fat, 3g saturated fat, 0 trans fat,
8g carbohydrates, 160mg cholesterol, 401mg sodium, 1g fiber

CHICKEN PICCATA
(MAKES 4 SERVINGS)

2 teaspoons extra-virgin olive oil
4 (3-ounce) skinless, boneless chicken breast fillets, lightly pounded
Salt and freshly ground pepper to taste
3 cloves fresh garlic, minced
1 cup low-sodium, fat-free chicken broth
2 tablespoons dry white wine
4 teaspoons lemon juice
1 tablespoon all-purpose flour
2 tablespoons chopped fresh parsley
1 tablespoon capers
Lemon wedges for garnish

Rinse chicken breast fillets under cold water and pat dry, then place breasts between layers of wax paper and lightly pound fillets with a meat mallet. Lightly sprinkle each fillet with salt and pepper if desired. Heat 1 teaspoon of olive oil in a large heavy-bottomed skillet over medium heat, add chicken fillets, and cook until fillets are lightly browned and centers cooked (juice will run clear). Transfer fillets to a serving platter and put in a low-temperature oven to keep warm. Add remaining teaspoon of oil and garlic to skillet and cook for 30 seconds to soften. Combine chicken broth, wine, lemon juice, and flour in skillet where chicken was cooked. Stir to blend, and continue stirring until mixture thickens. Add parsley and capers to sauce. Remove chicken from oven, place each fillet on a plate, and spoon mixture over fillets. Garnish with lemon wedges. Serve with cooked spinach linguine or pasta of choice.

Approx. 223 calories per serving
21g protein, 11g total fat, 2g saturated fat, 0 trans fat,
4g carbohydrates, 48mg cholesterol, 380mg sodium, <0.5g fiber

BROILED TUNA AND TOMATO
(MAKES 4 SERVINGS)

4 (3-ounce) tuna fillets
4 tablespoons extra-virgin olive oil
2 large cloves garlic, minced
1 tablespoon chopped parsley
Salt to taste
Freshly ground pepper to taste
1½ teaspoons white wine vinegar
8 (½-inch) slices fresh tomato
Italian parsley, chopped, for garnish

Rinse fillets, pat dry, and set aside. Combine in a covered container 2 tablespoons olive oil, garlic, parsley, salt and pepper. Add fillets, turning to coat well. Marinate fillets at room temperature for 2 hours. In another bowl, combine remaining olive oil, vinegar, and salt and pepper if desired. Arrange sliced tomatoes in a flat container in one layer and pour oil mixture over tomatoes; marinate at room temperature for 2 hours. Heat broiler, place tuna on grilling pan about 4 inches below heat, and broil each side of fillets for about 2–3 minutes. Arrange 2 slices of tomatoes on each plate; add tuna fillets to top of tomatoes and garnish with parsley. Serve while hot.

Approx. 224 calories per serving
20g protein, 18g total fat, 2.8g saturated fat, 0 trans fat,
2g carbohydrates, 38mg cholesterol, 35mg sodium, 0 fiber

SHRIMP IN SPICY BLACK BEAN SAUCE
(MAKES 4–6 SERVINGS)

2 jumbo cloves garlic, minced
2 tablespoons + 2 teaspoons extra-virgin olive oil
3 teaspoons chili powder
3 teaspoons cumin
2 cups canned black beans, rinsed and drained
1½ cups low-sodium, fat-free chicken broth
24 jumbo shrimp, peeled and deveined
Salt and freshly ground pepper to taste
Parsley, chopped for garnish

Sauté all but 2 teaspoons of garlic in 1 tablespoon of olive oil until almost browned. Add chili powder and cumin, and sauté for another minute. Add beans to garlic mixture, stirring frequently, and cook for another 3–4 minutes. Stir in chicken broth and transfer mixture to a food processor or blender. Puree mixture and return to skillet. Simmer sauce for 5 minutes, stirring often. Set aside, but keep warm. Rinse shrimp and pat dry; season with salt and pepper. Heat oil and sauté shrimp with remaining garlic. Cook until shrimp are lightly browned outside and cooked through inside, turning often. Remove shrimp from oil with a slotted spoon and set aside. Warm sauce and pour onto serving platter. Arrange shrimp on top of sauce and garnish with parsley. Serve immediately, with rice if desired.

Approx. 211 calories per serving
19g protein, 9g total fat, 1g saturated fat, 0 trans fat,
16g carbohydrates, 112mg cholesterol, 555mg sodium, 5g fiber

LEMONY CHICKEN AND VEGETABLES
(MAKES 4 SERVINGS)

3 tablespoons juice from fresh lemon halves
1 tablespoon fresh grated lemon peel
2 tablespoons extra-virgin olive oil
¼ teaspoon salt (optional)
¼ teaspoon freshly ground pepper
4 cloves garlic, freshly crushed
1 teaspoon paprika
1½ pounds skinless, boneless dark meat chicken
¾ pound yellow squash, quartered lengthwise
¾ pound zucchini, quartered lengthwise
¼ cup chopped fresh chives

Whisk together lemon juice, peel, oil, salt, and pepper. Reserve 2 tablespoons of mixture in a separate cup. Add to original mixture garlic and paprika and pour over chicken; marinate in a covered container in the refrigerator for 3–4 hours. When chicken is marinated, heat grill to medium-high heat. Remove chicken from marinade and place on grill along with squash, zucchini, and juiced lemon halves. Close grill top and cook for 10–12 minutes or until juices from chicken run clear when pierced. Turn chicken 1 time while grilling. Cook squash, zucchini, and lemon halves until tender and brown. Remove chicken from grill and cut into 1-inch-wide pieces. Cut squash and zucchini pieces in half. Place chicken and vegetables on a platter and pour reserved marinade over vegetables; sprinkle with chives. Garnish platter with grilled lemon halves and serve.

Approx. 255 calories per serving
29g protein, 15g total fat, 3g saturated fat, 0 trans fat,
8g carbohydrates, 105mg cholesterol, 254mg sodium, 2g fiber

HORSERADISH-ENCRUSTED SALMON
(MAKES 2 SERVINGS)

Olive oil cooking spray
2 (6-ounce) salmon fillets, skin intact
⅓ cup plain dried bread crumbs
1 tablespoon low-fat sour cream
2 tablespoons prepared fresh horseradish
2 tablespoons chopped fresh dill
Aged balsamic vinegar to drizzle (optional)

Lightly spray a shallow baking pan with cooking oil spray. Rinse fillets under cold water, pat dry with paper towels, and place skin side down in baking pan. In a food processor, combine bread crumbs, sour cream, horseradish, and dill. Pulse ingredients on low speed into a thick paste. Divide into 2 portions and top each fillet with mixture. Place fillets in oven and bake at 350 degrees until fillets flake easily and topping crusts to a golden brown (about 12–15 minutes). Serve hot, drizzle with a small amount of balsamic vinegar if desired.

Approx. 292 calories per serving
35g protein, 11g total fat, 2g saturated fat, 0 trans fat,
7g carbohydrates, 95mg cholesterol, 195mg sodium, 0 fiber

SALMON CAKES WITH SOUR CREAM DILL SAUCE
(MAKES 8 SERVINGS)

2 (14.75-ounce) cans of salmon
2 tablespoons extra-virgin olive oil
¾ cup chopped scallions
3 cloves fresh garlic, minced
½ teaspoon dried hot red pepper flakes
2 eggs
½ tablespoon lime juice
3 tablespoons cornstarch
Salt and freshly ground pepper to taste
1 cup fat-free or low-fat sour cream (optional)
4 tablespoons fresh dill, finely chopped (optional)

Drain and separate salmon; set aside. In a heavy-bottomed skillet over medium-low heat, add 2 teaspoons of oil, scallions, garlic, and pepper flakes. Sauté until scallions are soft, then set aside. In a bowl whisk together eggs, lime juice, cornstarch, and salt and pepper. Add egg mixture to scallion mixture and gently fold in salmon. Form salmon mixture into 8 cakes and refrigerate for about 30 minutes. Add remaining oil to a large skillet over medium-low heat and add chilled salmon cakes. Slowly sauté cakes for about 2–3 minutes on each side until heated through. Mix sour cream and dill together, and serve each salmon cake garnished with a tablespoon of sour cream and dill sauce if desired.

Approx. 251 calories per serving
24g protein, 15g total fat, 3g saturated fat, 0 trans fat,
3g carbohydrates, 134mg cholesterol, 397mg sodium, <0.5g fiber

ENCRUSTED RED SNAPPER AND DILL SAUCE
(MAKES 4 SERVINGS)

4 (5–6-ounce) red snapper fillets
Olive oil cooking spray
4 tablespoons fresh lemon juice
Freshly ground pepper to taste
4 tablespoons prepared spicy brown mustard
2 plum tomatoes, deseeded and chopped
½ medium green bell pepper, finely chopped
2 cloves fresh garlic, chopped
2 tablespoons freshly chopped parsley
½ cup plain bread crumbs
2 tablespoons melted trans fat–free canola/olive oil spread

For Dill Sauce:

2 tablespoons extra-virgin olive oil
2 tablespoons chopped shallots
1 tablespoon chopped fresh garlic
2 ounces dry white wine (not cooking wine)
2 tablespoons light cream cheese
2 tablespoons fat-free cream cheese
3 tablespoons trans fat–free canola/olive oil spread
4 tablespoons freshly chopped dill
Salt to taste (optional)
Generous dash of white pepper

Rinse fillets under cold water and pat dry with paper towels. Place fillets on a non-stick baking sheet lightly coated with cooking oil spray. Drizzle lemon juice over fillets and season with pepper to taste. Spread 1 tablespoon of mustard on each fillet. Combine tomatoes, green bell peppers, garlic, parsley, and bread crumbs; stir to mix well. Cover each fillet with vegetable bread crumb mixture and drizzle top of mixture with melted canola/olive oil spread. Bake for about 15 minutes at 350 degrees or until fillets flake easily and topping is lightly golden brown and crusty.

Dill Sauce:

Heat oil in a non-stick skillet over medium heat and sauté shallots and garlic until soft. Add wine and simmer on low heat, stirring often until mixture becomes slightly syrupy. Slowly fold in both cream cheeses and canola/olive oil spread, constantly stirring until melted. Add in dill and salt and pepper. Reduce heat to very low to keep warm until ready to serve. Drizzle sauce over and around sides of fillets.

Approx. 288 calories per serving without sauce
37g protein, 8g total fat, 2g saturated fat, 0 trans fat,
13g carbohydrates, 60mg cholesterol, 446mg sodium, 1g fiber

Approx. 359 calories per serving with sauce
38g protein, 15.5g total fat, 3.5g saturated fat, 0 trans fat,
13.5g carbohydrates, 63mg cholesterol, 523.5mg sodium, 0 fiber

ORANGE HORSERADISH-ENCRUSTED SCALLOPS
(MAKES 4 SERVINGS)

Olive oil cooking spray
1½ pounds sea scallops
⅓ cup plain dried bread crumbs
2 tablespoons prepared fresh horseradish
2 tablespoons freshly grated orange peel
1 tablespoon extra-virgin olive oil
Arugula leaves for garnish (optional)

Lightly spray the inside of a shallow oven-safe casserole dish with cooking spray. Place scallops in the casserole dish in a single layer. In a food processor, combine bread crumbs, horseradish, orange peel, and oil. Pulse ingredients on low speed into a thick paste. Spread mixture over the top of scallops and bake in a 350-degree oven until scallops are opaque and topping is a crusty golden brown (about 12–15 minutes). Divide into 4 portions and serve hot on a bed of arugula leaves if desired.

Approx. 180 calories per serving (about 8 scallops)
28g protein, 5g total fat, <0.5g saturated fat, 0 trans fat,
7g carbohydrates, 50mg cholesterol, 406mg sodium, <0.5g fiber

STEAMED DUNGENESS CRAB
(MAKES 2 SERVINGS)

*4 whole crab leg clusters (about 1½ pounds per cluster, fresh or frozen), large
   claws, cracked*
4 large cloves fresh garlic, halved
Scant sprinkle of accent seasoning (optional)
Scant sprinkle of garlic salt (optional)
Water enough to almost cover clusters
4 lemon wedges
Melted trans fat–free canola/olive oil spread for dipping (optional)

Place clusters in a large aluminum (turkey-sized) baking pan. Add garlic, accent seasoning, and garlic salt to taste if desired. Cover clusters with
water and cover pan tightly with foil. Bake covered at 450 degrees until
water begins to steam. Allow to steam for about 5 minutes, reduce heat to
250 degrees, and allow clusters to bathe in seasoned water about 15–20
minutes longer. Remove from oven, serve warm with lemon wedges and
melted canola/olive oil spread if desired.

Approx. 280 calories per serving
3g protein, 3g total fat, <0.5g saturated fat, 0 trans fat,
2g carbohydrates, 194mg cholesterol, 962mg sodium, 0 fiber

GRILLED WHOLE RAINBOW TROUT AND CHIVE SAUCE

(MAKES 4 SERVINGS)

4 (7–8-ounce) whole boneless trout with skin intact, cleaned and dressed
Garlic powder to taste
Freshly ground black pepper
Sea salt to taste (optional)
Olive oil cooking spray
⅓ cup light sour cheese
½ tablespoon water
4 teaspoons lime juice
⅛ teaspoon salt (optional)
⅛ teaspoon white pepper
3 tablespoons freshly chopped chives
Fresh spinach, sautéed (optional)

Turn on outdoor grill to high and close grill lid. Rinse trout under cold water and pat dry with paper towels. Season trout with garlic powder, pepper, and salt. Spray a cast-iron skillet with cooking oil spray and place skillet on grill. When skillet is hot, add fish. Turn trout over once to brown both sides and cook until meat flakes easily. While fish is browning combine sour cream, water, and lime juice in a small saucepan. Heat on low, stirring constantly, until blended, then add salt, pepper, and chives. Remove sauce from direct heat, but keep warm. When trout is ready, place each trout on a bed of sautéed spinach and spoon ⅛ cup of chive mixture over each trout. Serve immediately, while hot.

Approx. 309 calories per serving
50g protein, 10g total fat, 3.6g saturated fat, 0 trans fat,
2g carbohydrates, 138mg cholesterol, 239mg sodium, 0 fiber

BLACKENED TUNA STEAKS WITH MUSTARD GINGER SAUCE
(MAKES 4 SERVINGS)

4 (6-ounce) tuna steaks, about 1–1½ inches thick
½ cup light orange juice
4 cloves fresh garlic, chopped
1 teaspoon finely grated ginger
3 tablespoons low-sodium soy sauce
2 tablespoons sherry
1 tablespoon Dijon mustard
1 tablespoon honey
1 lemon, quartered

In a small bowl combine orange juice, garlic, ginger, soy sauce, sherry, mustard, and honey. Whisk for about 1 minute to blend marinade, then reserve and refrigerate ⅛ cup of marinade for basting tuna steaks during cooking. Rinse fish under cold water and pat dry with paper towels. Place fish in a single layer in a container and pour balance of marinade over fish. Put a tight-fitting lid on container and turn container over several times to allow marinade to coat all sides of fish. Refrigerate fish in marinade for 1–2 hours if possible, or for at least 30 minutes. When fish has marinated long enough, turn on outdoor grill to high and close grill lid. Spray a cast iron skillet with cooking oil spray and place skillet on grill. When skillet is very hot, remove fish from marinade container and place on hot skillet. Blacken fish on one side before turning over. Before turning, brush tops of fish generously with half of the reserved marinade. Turn over fish to blacken the other side and brush blackened side with the remainder of reserved marinade. Test centers and flakiness for desired doneness. Remove from heat and serve immediately.

Approx. 205 calories per serving
35g protein, 6g total fat, 1g saturated fat, 0 trans fat,
0 carbohydrates, 96mg cholesterol, 100mg sodium, 0 fiber

STUFFED SESAME CHICKEN BREASTS
(MAKES 4 SERVINGS)

4 (4–5-ounce) skinless, boneless chicken breasts
Salt and freshly ground pepper to taste
1 tablespoon dried tarragon or 4 sprigs fresh tarragon
½ red bell pepper, deseeded and thinly sliced
½ green bell pepper, deseeded and thinly sliced
4 tablespoons lime juice
¼ small red chili pepper, finely minced (optional)
¼ cup sesame seeds
Extra-virgin olive oil to drizzle
4 fresh tarragon sprigs for garnish

Rinse breasts under cold water and pat dry with paper towels. With a sharp knife, split open one side of breasts to create a pocket. Season inside of breasts with salt and pepper as desired and tarragon (¼ tablespoon of dried tarragon per breast or 1 full sprig stuffed inside the pocket of each breast). Insert slices of both red and green bell peppers into each breast pocket and then close, securing with a toothpick. Combine lime juice and chili pepper; set aside. Sprinkle each breast with a generous amount of sesame seeds and place breasts in a single layer on a non-stick baking sheet. Drizzle tops of breasts with lime/chili mixture and bake at 400 degrees for about 30 minutes, or until chicken is tender and cooked through. Set oven to broil, and lightly drizzle olive oil over the top of each breast. Place baking sheet under broiler and broil chicken breasts until sesame seeds are golden brown. Serve garnished with fresh sprigs of tarragon.

Approx. 237 calories per serving
37g protein, 8g total fat, 1g saturated fat, 0 trans fat,
4g carbohydrates, 96mg cholesterol, 85mg sodium, 1g fiber

BROILED MANGO CHICKEN BREAST FILLETS
(MAKES 4 SERVINGS)

4 (4–5-ounce) skinless, boneless chicken breast fillets
Salt and freshly ground pepper to taste
4 large bay leaves, crumbled
2 teaspoons finely chopped fresh garlic
6 large pitted black olives, halved
3 tablespoons of dry cream sherry
1 tablespoon extra-virgin olive oil
2 ripe but firm mangos, peeled and cut into wedges

Rinse fillets under cold water and pat dry with paper towels. Place fillets in a single layer in a shallow baking dish. Sprinkle tops of fillets with salt and pepper as desired. Scatter crumbled bay leaves, garlic, and olives over fillets. In a small bowl combine sherry and olive oil. Whisk to blend and drizzle over fillets. Scatter mango wedges over and around fillets. Place baking dish in oven and bake at 350 degrees for about 8–10 minutes, or until juices run clear when fillets are pierced with a fork. Set oven to broil. Transfer baking dish to top rack about 4 inches under heat and broil tops of fillets until lightly browned. Serve hot, drizzled with juices from baking dish and topped with pieces of mangos.

Approx. 297 calories per serving
36g protein, 8g total fat, 1g saturated fat, 0 trans fat,
18g carbohydrates, 96mg cholesterol, 86mg sodium, 1g fiber

BROILED SPICY TURKEY BURGERS
(MAKES 4 PATTIES)

1 pound freshly ground turkey breast
2 cloves fresh garlic, finely chopped
3 scallions, finely chopped
½ cup fresh spinach, chopped
½ cup Italian-seasoned bread crumbs
½ teaspoon red hot pepper sauce
½ teaspoon Worcestershire sauce
2 whole wheat pita loaves cut in half with pockets opened
Alfa sprouts, sliced tomato, lettuce, mustard, etc., as desired for garnish

Turn on oven broiler. In a large bowl, combine ground turkey, garlic, scallions, spinach, bread crumbs, hot pepper sauce, and Worcestershire sauce. Stir to mix thoroughly and form into 4 equal-size patties. Place patties on a broiler pan and place in oven about 4 inches under broiler. Broil burgers on each side for roughly 6 minutes, turning only once. Cook until centers are no longer pink. Remove from oven. Place each burger inside a pita pocket and garnish as desired.

Approx. 219 calories per patty
22g protein, 9g total fat, 3g saturated fat, 0 trans fat,
10g carbohydrates, 84mg cholesterol, 229mg sodium, <1g fiber

WHOLE WHEAT PENNE WITH SHRIMP AND BROCCOLI
(MAKES 4 SERVINGS)

8 ounces whole wheat penne
⅓ cup low-sodium, fat-free chicken broth
4 cloves fresh garlic, finely chopped
½ pound broccoli florets, cut into smaller florets
½ green bell pepper, diced
½ red bell pepper, diced
¼ cup diced scallions, white and green parts
¼ teaspoon hot red pepper flakes
16 ounces precooked baby shrimp
*½ cup Simple Tomato Pasta Sauce (page 362) or market-fresh tomato pasta
  sauce*
½ cup chopped fresh basil
Salt and freshly ground mixed pepper to taste
Grated Parmesan cheese for garnish, if desired

Bring water to a boil, add pasta, and cook pasta until *al dente*. Remove
from heat, drain pasta, and return to pot, drizzling with scant amount
of olive oil to keep pasta from sticking together. Set aside. While pasta
is cooking, heat chicken broth in a large skillet, and add garlic, broccoli,
green and red bell peppers, and scallions. Cover and cook vegetables over
medium-low heat until crispy tender. Reduce heat to low and add hot
pepper flakes and shrimp; stir to incorporate into vegetables and cook for
about 2–3 minutes. Add pasta sauce and cook for additional 2–3 minutes, stirring to mix well. Add penne to sauce and chopped basil. Toss to
coat pasta with sauce. Serve with a sprinkle of grated Parmesan cheese if
desired.

Approx. 315 calories per serving
28g protein, 3g total fat, 0.5g saturated fat, 0 trans fat,
42g carbohydrates, 75mg cholesterol, 605mg sodium, 5g fiber

BAKED FLOUNDER WITH CAPERS AND BABY SHRIMP
(MAKES 4 SERVINGS)

Olive oil cooking spray
8 (4-ounce) fillets of flounder
Scant amount of dried oregano
Scant amount of dried basil
Salt and freshly ground pepper to taste
20–24 cherry tomatoes, halved
4 teaspoons small capers, rinsed and drained
1 cup pre-cooked baby shrimp (defrosted and well drained)
6 tablespoons freshly grated Parmesan cheese
Scant amount of extra-virgin olive oil to drizzle
1 lemon, cut into 4 wedges for garnish

Lightly spray a shallow baking pan with cooking oil spray. Rinse fillets under cold water and pat dry. Place fillets in a single layer in baking pan, and add oregano, basil, and salt and pepper to taste. Scatter tomatoes, capers, and shrimp over fillets. Bake for about 8–10 minutes at 400 degrees. Remove from oven and turn oven to broil. Top fish with Parmesan cheese, drizzle a scant amount of olive oil over fish, and return to oven about 4 inches under broiler. Broil for about 15–20 seconds or until cheese lightly browns. Remove from oven and serve immediately, garnished with lemon wedges.

Approx. 272 calories per serving
53g protein, 5g total fat, 2g saturated fat, 0 trans fat,
<0.3g carbohydrates, 140mg cholesterol, 565mg sodium, 0 fiber

GRILLED TILAPIA
(MAKES 4 SERVINGS)

8 (4–5-ounce) tilapia fillets
Salt and freshly ground pepper to taste
Hot red pepper sauce to taste
Juice from 1 fresh lemon
Extra-virgin olive oil cooking spray
Fresh raw spinach for garnish

Rinse fillets under cold water and pat dry with paper towels. Place fillets on a large platter in a single layer, add salt and pepper to taste. Drizzle fillets with hot sauce and fresh lemon juice. Refrigerate fillets for at least 30 minutes. Turn on outdoor grill and set to high heat. Spray a cast iron skillet or grilling sheet lightly with olive oil spray, place on grill, and close grill top. Allow grill and skillet to reach 350–450 degrees. When skillet is hot enough, place fillets on skillet, seasoned side down, and close grill lid. Allow fillets to grill for about 4–5 minutes and then turn fillets over and allow other side to grill another 4–5 minutes or until fish turns opaque white. Remove from grill and serve hot on a bed of fresh spinach.

Approx. 200 calories per 2 fillets
42g protein, 5g total fat, 1g saturated fat, 0 trans fat,
2g carbohydrates, 110mg cholesterol, 120mg sodium, 0 fiber

BROILED GARLIC LAMB CHOPS
(MAKES 4 SERVINGS)

8 (4–5-ounce) lamb chops
4 cloves fresh garlic, finely chopped
½ tablespoon dried rosemary
Garlic salt to taste, if desired
3 tablespoons Dijon mustard
Juice from 1 lemon
1 tablespoon honey
2 tablespoons extra-virgin olive oil
¼ teaspoon red wine vinegar
Freshly ground pepper to taste
Fresh mint leaves for garnish

Set oven to broil. Rinse chops under cold water and pat dry with paper towels. Place them in a single layer on a broiling pan; set aside. Combine garlic and rosemary in a small bowl and mix. Vigorously rub garlic/rosemary mixture into both sides of chops, sprinkle with garlic salt if desired, and place chops about 4 inches under broiler. Broil to desired doneness. While chops are broiling, mix together mustard, lemon juice, honey, oil, vinegar, and pepper to taste, and blend well to incorporate ingredients. Remove chops from oven and place 2 chops on each serving plate. Spoon mustard mixture over chops, garnish with mint leaf, and serve immediately.

Approx. 574 calories per serving (2 chops)
68g protein, 24g total fat, 9g saturated fat, 0 trans fat,
6g carbohydrates, 216mg cholesterol, 192mg sodium, 0 fiber

TOMATO AND ANCHOVY SAUCE WITH PASTA
(MAKES 6–8 SERVINGS)

4 cloves garlic, finely chopped
3 tablespoons extra-virgin olive oil
10 anchovy fillets in olive oil
1 tablespoon finely chopped parsley
1 pound fresh tomatoes, peeled and chopped
Salt and freshly ground pepper to taste
1 pound dried whole grain pasta
¼ cup plain bread crumbs
¼ cup grated Romano cheese
Parsley sprigs for garnish

In a large skillet over medium-high heat, sauté garlic in oil until golden brown. Add in anchovy fillets and oil from anchovies. Crumble fillets into fine pieces to dissolve in oil. Add parsley, tomatoes, and salt and pepper to anchovy mixture and simmer for about 20–25 minutes. In boiling water, cook pasta to your liking and drain well. Lightly toss pasta with sauce and place on platter. In a separate bowl mix together bread crumbs and cheese. Top pasta with cheese mixture, garnish with parsley sprigs, and serve while hot.

Approx. 282 calories per serving
9g protein, 7g total fat, 2g saturated fat, 0 trans fat,
45g carbohydrates, 9mg cholesterol, 350mg sodium, 6g fiber

STEAMED MUSSELS WITH GARLIC AND DRY VERMOUTH
(MAKES 2 SERVINGS)

2 pounds fresh mussels, scrubbed and debearded (discard any open mussels)
1 tablespoon extra-virgin olive oil
3 cloves fresh garlic, minced
1 medium shallot, minced
1½ cups dry vermouth
1 cup low-sodium, fat-free chicken broth
Salt and freshly ground pepper to taste
1 tablespoon fresh lemon juice
Melted trans fat–free canola/olive oil spread (optional)
Lemon wedges for garnish

Keep cleaned mussels immersed in cold water until ready to steam. In a large skillet, heat oil and sauté garlic and shallots until tender, but do not brown. Add vermouth and chicken broth to skillet and stir to blend well with garlic mixture. With a slotted spoon, remove mussels from water and add to vermouth mixture. Add salt and pepper to taste, if desired. Cover skillet and increase heat to medium-high; steam mussels until all have opened, about 10 minutes. Reduce heat to very low to keep mussels warm until ready to serve, discarding any mussels which have not opened. To serve, remove mussels from skillet with a slotted spoon to individual serving bowls. Drizzle mussels with lemon juice and melted canola/olive oil spread, if desired. Garnish with lemon wedges and serve while hot.

Approx. 390 calories per serving (roughly 20–30 mussels)
54g protein, 10g total fat, 2g saturated fat, 0 trans fats,
17g carbohydrates, 127mg cholesterol, 1296mg sodium, 0 fiber

MEATLESS LASAGNA
(MAKES 6–8 SERVINGS)

1 pound dried whole grain lasagna noodles
3 cups sliced white mushrooms (about a 10-ounce box)
2½ tablespoons chopped fresh oregano
2½ teaspoons extra-virgin olive oil
2 large tomatoes (about 1½ pounds)
10 large pitted black olives, coarsely chopped
6 fresh garlic cloves, chopped
Salt and freshly ground pepper to taste
2 cups part-skim ricotta cheese
1 ounce grated Romano cheese
Freshly chopped basil for garnish

Cook pasta per package instructions. Meanwhile, in a large skillet over medium-high heat, add mushrooms, oregano, and olive oil. Sauté until mushrooms are tender; set aside. In a food processor or blender, process tomatoes until finely chopped. Add tomatoes and their juices, black olives, garlic, and salt and pepper to mushroom mixture and simmer covered for about 10 minutes. Drain pasta. In a large oven-safe casserole dish spread a thin layer of tomato and mushroom mixture, a layer of noodles, layer of ricotta cheese, followed by another layer of tomato and mushroom mixture, etc., until all of the ingredients are used. Finish with ricotta cheese. Top last layer of ricotta cheese with grated Romano cheese, followed by chopped basil. Place casserole in oven and bake for about 15–20 minutes, or until heated through. Remove from oven and serve while hot.

Approx. 318 calories per serving
9g protein, 1g total fat, <0.5g saturated fat, 0 trans fat,
40g carbohydrates, 0 cholesterol, 10mg sodium, 7g fiber

BLACK BEAN SEAFOOD BURGERS
(MAKES 6 PATTIES)

1 cup dry bulgur
1 cup hot water
1 tablespoon extra-virgin olive oil
2 tablespoons freshly chopped garlic
2 tablespoons freshly chopped white onion
Pinch of ground mixed pepper
1 cup fresh bay scallops
1 cup pre-cooked baby shrimp
1 can chopped clams, well drained
3 tablespoons chopped, deseeded plum tomatoes
¼ small hot pepper, finely chopped (optional)
1 cup canned black beans, well drained
½ cup egg substitute
Olive oil cooking spray
Salt and ground pepper to taste
Hot sauce (optional)
Lettuce leaves and slices of tomato for garnish

Place bulgur in a bowl, add hot water and cover, set aside until water has been absorbed (about 10 minutes). Heat oil in a large skillet; add garlic and onions, and sauté for about 2–3 minutes. Add a pinch of mixed pepper. Add scallops, and sauté until opaque in color. Add shrimp, clams, tomatoes, hot pepper, and beans; reduce heat to simmer, stir to blend flavors, and cook for another 3–4 minutes. Remove from heat and drain off any excess liquid. Transfer bean mixture to a large bowl, add bulgur and eggs, and stir to mix ingredients. Lightly spray a baking pan with cooking spray. Divide bean mixture into 6 portions and form into patties. Mixture will feel loose, but will come together while baking. Place patties on baking sheet, sprinkle with hot sauce, and salt and pepper to taste, and place into a 400-degree oven to bake for about 10–15 minutes. Set oven to broil and lightly brown tops of patties. Remove from oven and serve with lettuce leaves and slices of tomato.

Approx. 196 calories per patty
17g protein, 4g total fat, <0.5g saturated fat, 0 trans fat,
27g carbohydrates, 32mg cholesterol, 317mg sodium, 3g fiber

MOM'S TURKEY BURGERS
(MAKES 4 PATTIES)

1 pound freshly ground turkey breast
4 cloves fresh garlic, chopped
¼ cup egg substitute or 1 whole egg
*1 can (14 ounces) petite cut diced tomatoes with jalapeno peppers, well
    drained*
¼ cup plain bread crumbs
Salt and freshly ground pepper to taste

Preheat oven to broil. In a large mixing bowl, combine turkey, garlic,
egg, well-drained tomatoes (put tomatoes in a colander and press down
on them with a heavy spoon to drain off as much liquid as possible), bread
crumbs, and salt and pepper. Mix well to combine ingredients and form
into 4 patties. Place patties on a baking sheet about 4 inches below broiler. Broil each side 3–4 minutes or until tops are crusty and juices run clear
when pierced with a fork. Garnish as desired.

Approx. 283 calories per patty
23g protein, 17g total fat, 5g saturated fat, 0 trans fat,
0 carbohydrates, 85mg cholesterol, 75mg sodium, 0 fiber

FETTUCCINE WITH SMOKED SALMON AND BASIL PESTO
(MAKES 4 SERVINGS)

8 ounces dried whole grain fettuccine pasta
Drizzle of extra-virgin olive oil
¼ cup fresh Basil Pesto Sauce (page 357) or market-fresh pesto
10 pitted black olives, halved
½ tablespoon capers, rinsed well and drained
6 ounces nova smoked salmon (cut into thin strips)
1 tablespoon freshly grated Romano cheese
4 sprigs fresh basil leaves for garnish

Bring water to a boil, add pasta, and cook pasta until *al dente*. Remove from heat, drain pasta, and return to pot, drizzling with scant amount of olive oil to keep pasta from sticking together. Set aside. Meanwhile, warm pesto sauce in a saucepan under low heat, add olives and capers, remove from heat, and add salmon. In a large serving bowl, toss pasta with salmon mixture. Divide into 4 portions, and serve with ¼ tablespoon of cheese, garnished with a fresh basil sprig.

Approx. 323 calories per serving
15g protein, 10g total fat, 2g saturated fat, 0 trans fat,
44g carbohydrates, 14mg cholesterol, 540mg sodium, <1g fiber

BROILED HALIBUT STEAKS WITH TOMATO PESTO
(MAKES 4 SERVINGS)

4 (6-ounce) halibut steaks
Olive oil cooking spray
Salt and freshly ground pepper to taste
4 tablespoons market-fresh tomato pesto
4 lemon wedges for garnish

Preheat oven to broil. Rinse steaks under cold water and pat dry with paper towels. Lightly spray a broiler pan with olive oil spray and place steaks on pan. Season steaks with salt and pepper to taste, and place pan under broiler about 4 inches from heat. Cook 4–5 minutes per side or until steaks are opaque in color. Warm pesto in a small saucepan over low heat, stirring constantly. Place steaks on individual plates and top each steak with 1 tablespoon of pesto. Garnish with lemon wedge.

Approx. 261 calories per serving
46g protein, 6g total fat, <1g saturated fat, 0 trans fat,
2g carbohydrates, 69mg cholesterol, 275mg sodium, 0 fiber

CODFISH IN A SUNDRIED TOMATO PESTO SAUCE
(MAKES 4 SERVINGS)

4 medium tomatoes, chopped
4 cloves fresh garlic, chopped
¼ cup market-fresh sundried tomato pesto
1 tablespoon Sambuca
2 tablespoons chopped sundried tomatoes, drained
1 teaspoon capers, drained and well rinsed
10 Kalamata olives, halved
4 (6-ounce) fillets of cod
⅔ cup dry vermouth
1 bay leaf
¼ teaspoon peppercorns
Salt and freshly ground pepper to taste
4 lemon wedges for garnish
4 fresh parsley sprigs for garnish

In a heavy skillet, add tomatoes, garlic, pesto, Sambuca, sundried tomatoes, capers, and olives. Cook mixture over medium-low heat. Stir often to marry flavors. Reduce heat to low to keep sauce warm. In a separate
skillet, add cod, vermouth, bay leaf, peppercorns, and salt and pepper to
taste. Bring to a boil and reduce heat to simmer; cover and simmer for 10–
12 minutes or until fish is opaque in color and flakes easily. Meanwhile,
warm a platter in the oven at 175 degrees. When fish is ready, transfer to
warm platter and return platter to oven to keep fish warm. Drain liquid
from fish skillet through a strainer, add strained liquid to tomato pesto
sauce, and simmer for 2–3 minutes. Remove fish from oven and spoon
sauce over fish; garnish with lemon wedges and parsley sprigs. Serve immediately.

Approx. 214 calories per serving
39g protein, 3.8g total fat, 0.3g saturated fat, 0 trans fat,
10g carbohydrates, 54mg cholesterol, 441mg sodium, 2g fiber

TROUT ALMANDINE
(MAKES 4 SERVINGS)

4 (4-ounce) trout fillets
1½ tablespoons trans fat–free canola/olive oil spread, melted
3 tablespoons fresh lemon juice
½ teaspoon dried thyme
1 tablespoon finely chopped white onion
Salt to taste
Paprika to sprinkle
3 tablespoons finely chopped parsley
¼ cup sliced raw almonds
Canola oil cooking spray
4 lemon wedges for garnish

Rinse fillets under cold water and pat dry with paper towels. Combine melted canola/olive oil spread, lemon juice, thyme, onion, and salt in a small mixing bowl and whisk to blend flavors. Place fillets in a single layer in an oven-safe casserole dish and pour mixture over fish. Allow mixture to get under fillets as well. Top each fillet with paprika and parsley. Bake at 375 degrees for 12–15 minutes or until fish flakes easily and is opaque in color. Turn oven to broil. Top fish with almonds, and spray with a scant amount of cooking spray. Place fillets about 4 inches under broiler, and broil fillets for 2–3 minutes or until almonds are lightly toasted. Remove from broiler and serve immediately with lemon wedges.

Approx. 184 calories per serving
24g protein, 10g total fat, 1g saturated fat, 0 trans fat,
2g carbohydrates, 60mg cholesterol, 51mg sodium, 1g fiber

BROILED SCALLOPS WITH ORANGE GINGER SAUCE
(MAKES 4 SERVINGS)

Olive oil cooking spray
1½ pounds sea scallops
Salt and freshly ground pepper to taste
¼ of a fresh lime
Juice from 3 fresh oranges
¼ cup light mayonnaise
2 tablespoons prepared fresh horseradish
¼ teaspoon honey
¼ teaspoon ground ginger
1 tablespoon extra-virgin olive oil
Generous pinch of all-purpose flour

Spray a large oven-safe casserole dish with cooking spray. Place scallops in a single layer in casserole dish. Sprinkle scallops with salt and pepper to taste. Squeeze juice from ¼ of a fresh lime over scallops. Place casserole about 4 inches under broiler and broil scallops until opaque; turn scallops over after 3 minutes, and broil other side until also opaque in color. Remove from oven, set aside, and set oven to bake at 175 degrees. Combine orange juice, mayonnaise, horseradish, honey, ginger, olive oil, and salt and pepper in a small saucepan. Whisk to blend on low heat to a simmer. When sauce begins to simmer, whisk in flour. Cook for 1–2 minutes, whisking constantly until sauce is smooth. Add sauce to scallops and return to a slightly warm oven of 175 degrees for 3–4 minutes to allow sauce to thicken and marry flavors with scallops. Serve hot.

Approx. 210 calories per serving
29g protein, 6g total fat, 0.1g saturated fat, 0 trans fat,
13g carbohydrates, 57mg cholesterol, 389mg sodium, 0 fiber

CRAB PATTY BURGERS
(MAKES 4 PATTIES)

1 pound crab meat, well drained
¼ cup diced celery
1 tablespoon chopped green bell pepper
1 tablespoon chopped white onion
1 teaspoon Worcestershire sauce
1 teaspoon red hot pepper sauce (optional)
½ teaspoon salt (optional)
Dash of Old Bay seasoning
1 cup light mayonnaise
½ cup grated cheddar cheese
Scant amount of canola oil cooking spray
Lemon wedges for garnish

Mix all ingredients in a large bowl. Form into 4 patties and place on broiling sheet lightly sprayed with cooking oil. Place under broiler and broil for about 2 minutes, or until patties are lightly browned. Garnish with lemon wedges and serve.

Approx. 375 calories per patty
27g protein, 26g total fat, 5g saturated fat, 0 trans fat,
5g carbohydrates, 136mg cholesterol, 875mg sodium, 0.2g fiber

PAN-GRILLED GROUND PORK BURGERS
(MAKES 4 PATTIES)

Canola oil cooking spray
1½ pounds fresh lean ground pork
4 scallions, white and green parts, chopped
½ teaspoon garlic powder
½ teaspoon paprika
¼ teaspoon cayenne
Freshly ground pepper to taste
1 tablespoon chopped capers
Raw onion and stone-ground mustard for garnish (optional)

Lightly spray a stovetop ridged grill pan with cooking oil. Turn stovetop to high heat and preheat pan. Mix pork, scallions, spices, and capers together. Divide into 4 patties. When grill pan is very hot, place patties in pan, reduce heat to medium-high, and grill each side for about 4–5 minutes or until juices run clear, flipping patties only once. When completely cooked, serve garnished with sliced raw onion and stone-ground mustard.

Approx. 220 calories per patty
30g protein, 11g total fat, 4g saturated fat, 0 trans fat,
0 carbohydrates, 85mg cholesterol, 148mg sodium, 0 fiber

MUSSELS IN SPICY RED SAUCE
(MAKES 2 SERVINGS)

4 cloves fresh garlic, chopped
1 small onion, chopped
½ tablespoon extra-virgin olive oil
1 (28-ounce) can seasoned diced tomatoes
½ cup dry vermouth or other dry white wine
2 tablespoons low-sodium, low-fat chicken stock (optional)
1 teaspoon dry oregano
½ teaspoon Tabasco sauce, or to taste
Salt and freshly ground pepper to taste
1 large shallot, chopped
1 cup water
1 cup dry vermouth
40 small mussels in shells, scrubbed and debearded (about 1½–2 pounds)

In a large skillet, sauté garlic and onion in olive oil until soft; do not brown. Add tomatoes and juice, ½ cup vermouth, chicken stock, oregano, Tabasco, and salt and pepper to taste. Stir to blend flavors, bring to a boil, cover, reduce heat to low, and simmer for 15–20 minutes, stirring occasionally. Reduce heat to very low to keep sauce warm. In a large skillet, add shallots, water, 1 cup vermouth, and mussels. Cover skillet and bring to a boil. Reduce heat to simmer and cook until mussels open (5–8 minutes). Discard any mussels that do not open. With a slotted spoon, remove cooked mussels from steam pan and add to sauce. Remove 1 cup of steam broth with shallots included and add to sauce and mussels. Stir sauce to blend in broth and to cover mussels with sauce. Cover skillet and allow mixture to remain on low heat to keep warm for another 5–10 minutes while flavors marry. Divide mussels and sauce into 2 portions, and serve warm with crusty bread to sop up the sauce.

Approx. 240 calories per serving
16g protein, 6g total fat, 0.7g saturated fat, 0 trans fat,
20g carbohydrates, 35mg cholesterol, 770mg sodium, 2g fiber

GRILLED OR BAKED MUSSELS
(MAKES 2 SERVINGS)

1 large shallot, chopped
1 cup water
1 cup dry vermouth
40 small (about 2 pounds) mussels in shells, scrubbed and debearded
Extra-virgin olive oil to drizzle
2 cloves garlic, finely chopped
2 tablespoons chopped fresh parsley
½ cup plain bread crumbs
Salt and freshly ground pepper to taste
Lemon wedges for garnish
Tabasco sauce (optional)

In a large skillet, add shallots, water, vermouth, and mussels. Cover skillet and bring to boil. Reduce heat to simmer and cook until mussels open, about 5–8 minutes; discard any mussels that do not open. Remove mussels with a slotted spoon to a baking tray. Drizzle opened shells with a small amount of olive oil, sprinkle with chopped garlic, parsley, bread crumbs, and salt and pepper to taste. Bake at 350 degrees for about 8–10 minutes or until bread crumbs are golden brown, or grill on a medium-high heat grill (grilling may take a little longer). Divide into two portions and serve with lemon wedges, Tabasco sauce, and crusty bread if desired.

Approx. 126 calories per serving
14g protein, 2g total fat, 0.5g saturated fat, 0 trans fat,
12g carbohydrates, 35mg cholesterol, 336mg sodium, 0 fiber

SPINACH FETTUCCINE WITH BABY ARTICHOKES

(MAKES 4 SERVINGS)

8 ounces dried spinach fettuccine
9-ounce package baby artichokes, thawed
3 tablespoons extra-virgin olive oil
6 cloves fresh garlic, finely chopped
16 large raw shrimp, peeled and deveined
½ cup dry vermouth
2 large plum tomatoes, finely chopped
1 cup low-sodium, fat-free chicken broth
12 pitted black olives, halved
1½ tablespoons trans fat–free canola/olive oil spread
1 teaspoon fresh lemon peel, finely grated
Salt to taste (optional)
½ teaspoon ground nutmeg
1 tablespoon chopped fresh parsley
Lemon wedges for garnish

Cook pasta per box directions, then remove from heat, drain pasta, and return to pot, drizzling with scant amount of olive oil to keep pasta from sticking together. Set aside. Cut artichokes lengthwise and remove outer leaves, cut off bases, and trim off tops about ⅓ way down. Remove fuzzy choke inside, discard, and cut remaining choke in half again. Repeat procedure until all chokes are cleaned and quartered. In a large skillet, add 2 tablespoons of oil and garlic, and sauté for 1 minute; add artichokes and cook for another 1–2 minutes. Add shrimp and vermouth; continue cooking, stirring often, until shrimp are pink. Add tomatoes, broth, olives, canola/olive oil spread, peel, salt, nutmeg, and pasta. Toss to coat pasta with sauce. Heat mixture till warmed through. Stir in parsley and drizzle with remaining olive oil. Serve with lemon wedges for garnish.

Approx. 437 calories per serving
17g protein, 17g total fat, 3g saturated fat, 0 trans fat,
51g carbohydrates, 43mg cholesterol, 195mg sodium, 2g fiber

ROSEMARY ROASTED CHICKEN BREASTS
(MAKES 4 SERVINGS)

4 chicken breasts with rib bones and skin (about 9–12 ounces each)
Salt and freshly ground pepper to taste
2 tablespoons trans fat–free canola/olive oil spread (room temperature)
3 teaspoons freshly minced rosemary leaves
3 cloves garlic, finely chopped
1 teaspoon fresh lemon zest
Extra-virgin olive oil to drizzle

Rinse breasts under cold water and pat dry, then remove any excess fat. Sprinkle rib bone sides of breasts with salt and pepper to taste and place breasts rib side down on broiler pan. With a sharp pointed knife, insert blade into one end of skin and gradually slide blade under skin to create a pocket between skin and breast meat. In a small bowl combine canola/olive oil spread, rosemary, garlic, and zest. Stir to blend flavors and textures. Divide into 4 portions. Use a small flat knife to stuff rosemary mixture under skin into pockets of chicken breasts. With a finger, gently press on the skin to spread out rosemary mixture over the breast meat inside the pocket (the skin pocket will allow the rosemary mixture and flavors to soak into the meat as the chicken bakes). Sprinkle the tops of each breast with freshly ground pepper and a drizzle of olive oil. Place broiler pan in oven and bake breasts for about 40–45 minutes at 450 degrees, on rack placed in center of oven. Remove from oven and peel off skin before serving if desired.

Approx. 233 calories per serving (with skin on)
29g protein, 12g total fat, 3.4g saturated fat, 0 trans fat,
0 carbohydrates, 83mg cholesterol, 109mg sodium, 0 fiber

CHICKEN AND SPICY HUMMUS
(MAKES 4 SERVINGS)

¼ cup olive oil

1 tablespoon finely chopped garlic

½ teaspoon ground cumin

½ teaspoon freshly ground black pepper

1½ pounds skinless boneless chicken breast, cut into 2-inch cubes

1 red bell pepper, sliced lengthwise into 1-inch wide strips

1 yellow banana pepper, sliced lengthwise into 1-inch wide strips

1 red onion, cut into strips

Salt to taste

4 lemon wedges for garnish

½ cup prepared spicy hummus

Combine oil, garlic, cumin, black pepper, chicken, red and yellow peppers, and salt in a Ziploc bag. Toss all ingredients until chicken is well coated with oil and seasonings. Line a broiler pan with tinfoil and spread chicken mixture out in a single layer. Place pan 4–6 inches under heat and broil ingredients for roughly 8–10 minutes, stirring once, until chicken is cooked through and veggies are lightly blackened. Divide hummus and chicken mixture each into 4 equal portions. Place hummus on plate and top with chicken mixture. Garnish plate with lemon wedge and serve with toasted pita wedges if desired.

Approx. 435 calories per serving
43g protein, 22g total fat, 3g saturated fat, 0 trans fat,
17g carbohydrates, 96mg cholesterol, 281mg sodium, 2g fiber

TURKEY MEATBALLS WITH WHOLE GRAIN PASTA AND TOMATO SAUCE

(MAKES 4 SERVINGS)

1½ pounds lean ground turkey breast
½ cup finely diced onion
1⅓ cups finely diced celery
2 tablespoons finely diced green bell pepper
1 tablespoon dry Italian seasoning mix
4 cloves fresh garlic, finely chopped
3 cups bread crumbs
½ cup liquid egg substitute
Salt and freshly ground pepper to taste
Olive oil cooking spray
8 ounces cooked whole grain spaghetti
2 cups Simple Tomato Pasta Sauce (page 362) or market-fresh tomato pasta
  sauce

In a large bowl combine ground turkey, onions, celery, green bell pepper, Italian seasoning, garlic, bread crumbs, egg, and salt and pepper. Mix well to combine ingredients and form into 12 meatballs. Heat a large skillet sprayed with a small amount of olive oil; reduce heat to medium-low and add meatballs. Cook turning often until meatballs are completely cooked, and outsides lightly browned. Serve with pasta and sauce.

Approx. 279 calories per serving
10g protein, 7.5g total fat, 0.8g saturated fat, 0 trans fat,
55g carbohydrates, 11mg cholesterol, 8mg sodium, 1g fiber

CALAMARI IN SPICY RED SAUCE
(MAKES 4–6 SERVINGS)

3 cups low-sodium canned tomato sauce
1 (28-ounce) can peeled Italian tomatoes, broken into pieces
1 cup Chianti wine
2 tablespoons freshly squeezed lemon juice
1 tablespoon extra-virgin olive oil
3 cloves garlic, chopped
1 small onion, chopped
1 teaspoon black pepper
Salt to taste (optional)
½ teaspoon cayenne pepper
6 fresh basil leaves, chopped
⅓ cup grated Romano cheese
2 pounds cleaned calamari, cut in ½-inch rings

In a large deep skillet, add tomato sauce, tomato pieces, wine, lemon juice, olive oil, garlic, onion, black pepper, salt to taste, cayenne, basil, and cheese. Simmer on medium-low heat for about 30 minutes to allow alcohol to burn off and infuse other ingredients with its flavor. Add calamari rings and continue to simmer for an additional 20–30 minutes, stirring occasionally. Calamari is cooked when it plumps and becomes opaque in color. Do not overcook calamari; it becomes tough. Serve with cooked fettuccine if desired.

Approx. 224 calories per serving
26g protein, 5g total fat, 0.7g saturated fat, 0 trans fat,
16g carbohydrates, 186mg cholesterol, 306mg sodium, 3g fiber

BLACK BEANS AND BROWN RICE
(MAKES 4–6 SERVINGS)

1½ cups dry black beans

5 cups water or low-sodium, fat-free chicken broth

2 bay leaves

1 teaspoon black pepper

Salt to taste

2 cloves garlic, chopped

1 medium onion, chopped

1 medium green bell pepper, chopped

½ teaspoon cayenne pepper

10 green Manzanilla olives, pitted and halved

1 tablespoon extra-virgin olive oil

½ cup Edmundo cooking wine or a dry white wine

3 cups cooked brown rice

Raw chopped onion for garnish

Wash beans under cold running water. Place beans, water or broth, and bay leaves in a large heavy-bottomed pot and bring to a boil. Boil for about 2–3 minutes. Remove from heat, cover, and soak beans for 1 hour. Add black pepper, salt to taste, garlic, onions, and bell peppers, bring to boil, then reduce heat to simmer, cover, and cook until beans are tender (about 1–1½ hours), adding extra water or broth if needed. When beans are tender, add cayenne pepper, olives, olive oil, and wine. Cook on simmer for roughly 20–30 minutes to allow alcohol to evaporate and flavors to marry. Serve over brown rice, and garnish with raw chopped onion.

Approx. 350 calories per serving (with chicken broth)
17g protein, 6g total fat, 0.57g saturated fat, 0 trans fat,
57g carbohydrates, 2mg cholesterol, 250mg sodium, 8g fiber

Approx. 321 calories per serving (with water)
13g protein, 4g total fat, 0.57g saturated fat, 0 trans fat,
56g carbohydrates, <1mg cholesterol, 250mg sodium, 8g fiber

LENTIL STEW
(MAKES 6–8 SERVINGS)

1½ cups dry lentils
1 medium onion, chopped
4 cloves garlic, chopped
1 tablespoon extra-virgin olive oil
5 cups low-sodium fat-free chicken broth
1 tablespoon Worcestershire sauce
1 (15-ounce) can diced tomatoes and juice
1 bay leaf
½ teaspoon thyme
½ teaspoon cayenne
¼ teaspoon ground pepper
Salt to taste
2 large potatoes, peeled and chopped
4 medium carrots, chopped
1 (10-ounce) bag fresh spinach
Dollop low-fat sour cream for garnish (optional)

Rinse lentils and set aside. In a large deep skillet, sauté onions and garlic in olive oil until tender but not browned. Add lentils, chicken broth, Worcestershire sauce, tomatoes, bay leaf, thyme, cayenne, ground pepper, and salt to taste. Bring to a boil, cover, and reduce to simmer for 20 minutes. Add potatoes, carrots, and spinach, and stir to incorporate all ingredients. Bring to a boil, cover, reduce to medium-high, and cook for 20–30 minutes or until lentils and vegetables are tender and most of the liquid has been absorbed. Remove bay leaf and serve stew garnished with a dollop of sour cream and a multigrain crusty bread if desired.

Approx. 215 calories per serving
15g protein, 3.3g total fat, 0.3g saturated fat, 0 trans fat,
36g carbohydrates, 1mg cholesterol, 123mg sodium, 7g fiber

GRILLED BLACKENED SALMON
(MAKES 4 SERVINGS)

1 teaspoon sea salt
1 tablespoon paprika
1 teaspoon onion powder
1 teaspoon garlic powder
1 teaspoon cayenne pepper
1 teaspoon mixed pepper flakes
½ teaspoon dried thyme
½ teaspoon dried basil
⅛ cup olive oil
4 (6–7-ounce) salmon fillets

Place a dry cast iron skillet on grill and heat to 400 degrees. Mix all seasonings together. Brush both sides of fillets with scant amount of olive oil and drench both sides in seasonings. Place fillets on hot skillet and blacken each side about 3–4 minutes or until blackened and fish flakes easily.

Approx. 426 calories per serving
34g protein, 19g total fat, 0.9g saturated fat, 0 trans fat,
3g carbohydrates, 130mg cholesterol, 240mg sodium, 0.7g fiber

ANGEL HAIR WITH FRESH MARINARA
(MAKES 6–8 SERVINGS)

16 ounces dried whole grain angel hair pasta
4 tablespoons extra-virgin olive oil
½ white onion, chopped
6 cloves fresh garlic, chopped
1 (28-ounce) can crushed Italian tomatoes
1 (6-ounce) can tomato paste
4–5 chopped fresh basil leaves
4 tablespoons freshly chopped parsley
1 teaspoon crushed red pepper flakes
Salt and freshly ground pepper to taste
½ cup white wine (optional)
Grated Parmesan cheese (optional)

Bring water to a boil, add pasta, and cook pasta until *al dente*. Remove from heat, drain pasta, and return to pot, drizzling with scant amount of olive oil to keep pasta from sticking together. Set aside. Heat oil in a heavy-bottomed skillet and sauté garlic and onion, but do not brown. Reduce heat to simmer. Add crushed tomatoes and tomato paste, basil, parsley, red pepper flakes, salt and pepper, and wine, and simmer for 30–40 minutes, stirring occasionally. Serve sauce over pasta sprinkled with cheese if desired.

Approx. 310 calories per serving
9.2g protein, 8.6g total fat, 0.8g saturated fat, 0 trans fat,
48g carbohydrates, 0 cholesterol, 246mg sodium, 6.6g fiber

LEMON SHRIMP PASTA
(MAKES 4–6 SERVINGS)

30–36 large shrimp, peeled and deveined
Juice from 4 fresh lemons
1 teaspoon lemon pepper
12 ounces bow tie pasta
1 tablespoon extra-virgin olive oil
4 cloves fresh garlic, chopped
4 scallions, white and green parts, sliced
10 black olives, pitted and coarsely chopped
⅛ teaspoon red hot pepper flakes
1 teaspoon ground garlic powder
3 tablespoons trans fat–free canola/olive oil spread
Salt to taste (optional)
Grated Parmesan cheese for garnish (optional)

Place shrimp in a large Ziploc bag and add lemon juice and lemon pepper. Allow shrimp to marinate in refrigerator for at least 30 minutes. Bring water to a boil, add pasta, and cook pasta until *al dente*. Remove from heat, drain pasta, and return to pot, drizzling with scant amount of olive oil to keep pasta from sticking together. Set aside. In a large skillet add olive oil, garlic, and scallions, and sauté lightly until soft. Add black olives and hot pepper flakes, then set aside, but keep warm. When shrimp has marinated, add shrimp, lemon juice, and garlic powder to scallion mixture. Bring to a low simmer and cook until shrimp are pink and cooked through. Add pasta, canola/olive oil spread, and salt to taste to shrimp mixture, and allow spread to melt while tossing pasta and lemon shrimp mixture to blend flavors. Serve hot with a sprinkle of Parmesan cheese if desired.

Approx. 326 calories per serving
16g protein, 9.5g total fat, 1.7g saturated fat, 0 trans fat,
42.2g carbohydrates, 64.5mg cholesterol, 232mg sodium, 0.4g fiber

GRILLED WHOLE SEA BASS
(MAKES 4 SERVINGS)

2 (1½-pound) sea bass, dressed and gutted
1 sprig fresh rosemary
½ of a fresh lemon, thinly sliced
Olive oil
¼ teaspoon garlic powder
¼ teaspoon onion powder
Lemon pepper seasoning to taste

For Sauce:

1 teaspoon sea salt (optional)
2 teaspoons capers, drained
4 cloves fresh garlic, crushed
4 tablespoons water
3 sprigs fresh rosemary
2 fresh bay leaves
1 teaspoon lime juice
2 tablespoons extra-virgin olive oil
Freshly ground pepper to taste

Wash fish and pat dry with paper towel, then place 1 sprig of rosemary and ½ of lemon slices (divided) in the cavity of each fish. Drizzle a small amount of olive oil over each fish and sprinkle with garlic powder, onion powder, and lemon pepper seasoning. Grill for about 5 minutes on each side or until fish is cooked through. Drizzle with sauce and serve garnished with remaining lemon slices.

Sauce:

In a food processor add salt, capers, garlic, and water; process until smooth. In a bowl crush rosemary and bay leaves. Add crushed bay leaf mixture and lime juice to garlic mixture. Stir in olive oil and ground pepper, and mix to blend.

Approx. 388 calories per serving
63g protein, 17g total fat, 2.9g saturated fat, 0 trans fat,
0 carbohydrates, 140mg cholesterol, 801mg sodium, 0 fiber

VEAL SCALOPPINE
(MAKES 4 SERVINGS)

1 pound (16 ounces) boneless veal, trimmed of excess fat
Salt and freshly ground pepper to taste
Olive oil cooking spray

For Sauce:

¼ cup low-sodium, fat-free chicken broth
½ cup chopped white onion
4 cloves fresh garlic, finely chopped
1 (12-ounce) can diced Italian herb tomatoes
4 tablespoons dry white wine
½ teaspoon dried oregano
6 anchovies, drained and broken into pieces
1 tablespoon capers, drained

Divide veal into 4 pieces. Place pieces one at a time between two pieces of wax paper. Starting from center, pound pieces with a meat mallet, working your way toward the edges, until the meat is about ⅛ of an inch in thickness. Season lightly with salt and pepper and set aside. Repeat procedure with all remaining pieces. Spray a large heavy skillet with cooking spray and heat over medium-high heat. Add veal pieces to skillet and cook for 2–4 minutes, turning fillets over once, until they reach desired doneness. Place fillets on a platter and cover with sauce. Serve warm.

Sauce:

Put chicken broth in a medium saucepan, add onions and garlic, and cook until tender. Stir in tomatoes, wine, oregano, anchovies, and capers. Cover pan and bring to a quick boil; reduce to very low heat, then simmer uncovered for 5–10 minutes.

Approx. 202 calories per serving
26g protein, 3.3g total fat, 0.98g saturated fat, 0 trans fat,
13.7g carbohydrates, 96mg cholesterol, 768mg sodium, 2g fiber

SPICY EGGPLANT
(MAKES 6–8 SERVINGS)

4 tablespoons extra-virgin olive oil
1 (1-pound) eggplant, thinly sliced (about ⅛-inch thick)
½ cup liquid egg substitute
¼ cup all-purpose flour
2 tablespoons finely minced fresh garlic
Salt and freshly ground pepper to taste
Cholula hot sauce or other spicy red hot sauce to taste
1½ cups fresh marinara sauce

Heat 1 tablespoon of oil in heavy-bottomed skillet over medium-high heat. Dip eggplant slices in eggs and then lightly into flour. Sprinkle slices with garlic, and salt and pepper to taste. Cook, adding only as much oil as needed, until golden brown, and transfer to warmed plate. Repeat until all eggplant slices are cooked. Layer cooked eggplant in an oven-safe casserole dish and drizzle each layer with a small amount of hot sauce and fresh marinara sauce. Repeat layers until all eggplant is used. Do not overdo sauces! Keep in 175-degree oven until ready to serve.

Approx. 117 calories per serving
1g protein, 10g total fat, 2g saturated fat, 0 trans fat,
3g carbohydrates, 0 cholesterol, 212mg sodium, 1g fiber

Side Dishes

SAFFRON RICE
(MAKES 4–6 SERVINGS)

3–4 cups low-sodium, fat-free vegetable broth
1 tablespoon extra-virgin olive oil
4 tablespoons chopped shallots
2 cloves garlic, minced
1 cup uncooked short-grain rice
1 cup dry white wine
¼ teaspoon crushed saffron threads
½ teaspoon dried thyme
Salt and freshly ground pepper to taste

Bring broth to a boil, then reduce heat to a low simmer. In a large skillet, heat olive oil, add shallots and garlic, and sauté until soft (about 5 minutes). Add rice and continue to sauté, stirring constantly to keep mixture from burning. Add wine, saffron, and thyme, stirring constantly, scraping in any brown bits from pan. When wine is absorbed, slowly add simmering broth, stirring constantly as broth is absorbed and rice has become tender (about 15–20 minutes). It's possible some of the broth will be left over. Add salt and pepper to taste.

Approx. 282 calories per serving
5g protein, 2g total fat, 0.34g saturated fat, 0 trans fat,
49g carbohydrates, 0 cholesterol, 87mg sodium, 2g fiber

ZESTY LEMON SWISS CHARD
(MAKES 4–6 SERVINGS)

1¼ pounds Swiss chard, cleaned and trimmed
2 tablespoons fresh lemon juice
1½ teaspoons extra-virgin olive oil
1 tablespoon lemon pepper
Salt to taste
½ cup golden raisins
2 tablespoons pine nuts

Shred Swiss chard into thin strips and place in a large bowl. Combine lemon juice, olive oil, lemon pepper, and salt; mix well with whisk. Drizzle over chard and toss. Add raisins and pine nuts, and toss. Let stand for 15 minutes before serving.

Approx. 120 calories per serving
2g protein, 5g total fat, 0.7g saturated fat, 0 trans fat,
21g carbohydrates, 0 cholesterol, 302mg sodium, 1g fiber

ORZO WITH FETA CHEESE AND BROCCOLI FLORETS
(MAKES 8 SERVINGS)

2 cups broccoli florets
3 cups low-sodium, fat-free chicken broth
8 ounces uncooked orzo (about 1 cup)
6 ounces feta cheese

In boiling water, cook broccoli florets until crispy tender. Drain, set aside, and keep warm. In a saucepan, bring chicken broth to a boil, reduce heat, add orzo, and cook until liquid is absorbed. Stir often to keep from burning. Fluff orzo with fork and add feta cheese, stirring to blend together. Transfer orzo to serving platter and top with broccoli florets.

Approx. 174 calories per serving
8g protein, 7g total fat, 3g saturated fat, 0 trans fat,
22g carbohydrates, 195mg cholesterol, 237mg sodium, 0 fiber

ROASTED PEPPERS
(MAKES 4–6 SERVINGS)

4 large red bell peppers
2 cloves garlic, peeled and sliced
4 tablespoons extra-virgin olive oil
Salt and freshly ground pepper to taste

Clean peppers and pat dry. Place peppers on moderately hot grill or on a rack under a broiler 1–2 inches from heat, turning often until skin is charred and blistered. Charring of entire skin takes about 15–20 minutes. Remove from grill or broiler and place peppers aside to cool. When cool enough to handle, rub off blackened skins. Cut each pepper in half, remove stalk and seeds, and cut into ½-inch strips. Place strips in a bowl, and add garlic, oil, and salt and pepper to taste. Toss and set aside for about 30 minutes before serving.

Approx. 108 calories per serving
1g protein, 10g total fat, 1g saturated fat, 0 trans fat,
7g carbohydrates, 0 cholesterol, 2mg sodium, 2g fiber

CLASSIC SPINACH AND PINE NUTS
(MAKES 4 SERVINGS)

¼ cup golden raisins
4 tablespoons pine nuts
2 tablespoons extra-virgin olive oil
4 cloves garlic, chopped
1½ (10-ounce) bags fresh spinach, cleaned
Fresh lemon juice
Extra-virgin olive oil to taste
Salt and freshly ground pepper to taste

Place raisins in a bowl and cover with boiling water. Let stand for approximately 10 minutes, until raisins are plump; drain well. In a skillet over medium heat, toast pine nuts, stirring constantly for about 1–2 minutes. Remove from heat, and set aside. In a large skillet, warm olive oil. Add garlic and sauté for 1–2 minutes, until golden. Add spinach a little at a time until it all becomes wilted (about 3–5 minutes), stirring constantly. Pour raisins over spinach and mix well. With a slotted spoon, transfer spinach to a serving dish, and sprinkle pine nuts over top. Serve immediately or, if serving at room temperature, add fresh lemon juice, and extra-virgin olive oil and salt and pepper to taste.

Approx. 149 calories per serving
4g protein, 12g total fat, 2g saturated fat, 0 trans fat,
10g carbohydrates, 0 cholesterol, 41mg sodium, 2g fiber

CHILLED STUFFED PASTA SHELLS
(MAKES 4 SERVINGS)

1 cup (canned) hearts of palm, chopped and well drained
1 cup chopped zucchini
2 cloves fresh garlic, finely minced
8 large pitted black olives, chopped
2 tablespoons chopped fresh parsley
2 tablespoons + 2 teaspoons extra-virgin olive oil
4 teaspoons freshly squeezed lemon juice
Salt and freshly ground pepper to taste
12 jumbo pasta shells, cooked al dente and drained
4 cups mixed salad greens

Combine hearts of palm, zucchini, garlic, olives, and parsley in a large bowl. Whisk together olive oil, lemon juice, and salt and pepper for vinaigrette. To bowl of vegetables, add 2 tablespoons of vinaigrette; gently mix. Stuff shells with vegetable mixture, cover, and refrigerate until well chilled. Refrigerate remaining vinaigrette. To serve, divide greens into 4 equal portions, top each serving with 3 stuffed shells, and drizzle with remaining vinaigrette.

Approx. 210 calories per serving
5g protein, 11g total fat, 1.4g saturated fat, 0 trans fat,
24g carbohydrates, 0 cholesterol, 255mg sodium, 2g fiber

GREEK RICE
(MAKES 4 SERVINGS)

1 cup short-grain rice
2 cups low-sodium vegetable broth
1 tablespoon extra-virgin olive oil
2 teaspoons minced garlic
2 tablespoons finely chopped onions
5 ounces fresh spinach, cleaned and chopped
¼ teaspoon dried oregano
Salt and freshly ground pepper to taste
¼ cup crumbled feta cheese
1 tablespoon lemon juice

Bring rice in vegetable broth to boil, cover tightly, reduce heat to simmer, and cook until liquid is absorbed. While rice is cooking, heat oil over medium-high heat and sauté garlic and onion until golden. Reduce heat to medium; add spinach a little at a time to allow spinach to wilt while mixing in garlic. When spinach is wilted, mix in oregano and salt and pepper to taste. Remove spinach mixture from heat, and add cooked rice, cheese, and lemon juice; toss well.

Approx. 255 calories per serving
12.5g protein, 5.7g total fat, 1.3g saturated fat, 0 trans fat,
22g carbohydrates, 5mg cholesterol, 146mg sodium, 1g fiber

GARLIC RICE
(MAKES 4 SERVINGS)

½ tablespoon extra-virgin olive oil
4 cloves fresh garlic, minced
1 cup basmati long-grain rice
2 cups low-sodium, fat-free chicken broth
¼ cup grated Parmesan cheese
2 tablespoons chopped fresh parsley
3 jumbo cloves roasted garlic, cut into small pieces
Salt and freshly ground pepper to taste
Fresh chopped parsley or cilantro for garnish

In a skillet, heat oil and sauté fresh garlic until golden brown. Bring rice in chicken broth to a boil, cover tightly, reduce heat to simmer, and cook until liquid is absorbed. Remove rice from heat, and add oil and sautéed garlic, cheese, parsley, roasted garlic, and salt and pepper to taste; toss well. Garnish with parsley or cilantro and serve.

Approx. 194 calories per serving
5g protein, 3g total fat, 0.3g saturated fat, 0 trans fat,
38g carbohydrates, 0 cholesterol, 3mg sodium, 1g fiber

COUSCOUS, TOMATOES, AND BLACK BEANS
(MAKES 4–6 SERVINGS)

1½ cups low-sodium vegetable broth

1 cup uncooked couscous

1 tablespoon extra-virgin olive oil

2 cloves garlic, minced

¼ cup fresh lemon juice

¼ teaspoon freshly ground pepper

1½ cups canned black beans, rinsed and drained

4 large plum tomatoes, chopped

½ cup red onion, finely chopped

Fresh parsley, finely chopped for garnish

In a saucepan, bring broth to a boil. Stir in couscous, remove from heat, cover, and let stand until liquid is absorbed. In a small skillet over medium heat, add olive oil and garlic, and sauté until golden brown. Remove sauté pan from heat, add lemon juice and pepper, and mix ingredients through. Transfer couscous to a large serving bowl. Fluff grains with fingers to separate. Add in garlic mixture, black beans, tomatoes, and chopped onions; stir gently to mix. Garnish with parsley and serve.

Approx. 210 calories per serving
8g protein, 3g total fat, 0.3g saturated fat, 0 trans fat,
37g carbohydrates, 0 cholesterol, 239mg sodium, 5g fiber

BROCCOLI WITH FRESH GARLIC

(MAKES 4–6 SERVINGS)

10–12 fresh broccoli spears, roughly 6 inches long
3 cups low-sodium, fat-free chicken broth
3 tablespoons extra-virgin olive oil
2–3 cloves fresh garlic, crushed
2 tablespoons chopped fresh parsley
Salt to taste
Pinch of freshly ground pepper to taste

Cook spears in a large skillet of chicken broth until slightly under-cooked (about 7 minutes). Test with a fork; do not overcook. Drain well and set aside. Heat oil in a large skillet over medium-high heat; add garlic and sauté until golden brown. Add broccoli, parsley, and seasonings to taste. Turn broccoli several times, mixing well with seasonings, oil, and garlic. Serve immediately.

Approx. 161 calories per serving
11g protein, 9g total fat, 2g saturated fat, 0 trans fat,
16g carbohydrates, 1mg cholesterol, 80mg sodium, 9g fiber

CRISPY TENDER RATATOUILLE
(MAKES 8 SERVINGS)

2 large eggplants, rinsed and cut into 1½-inch cubes
3 red bell peppers
¾ cup extra-virgin olive oil
2 large onions, chopped
8 garlic cloves, minced
4 small zucchini, cut to 1½-inch cubes
4 large ripe tomatoes, cored and diced
1 cup dry red wine
1 tablespoon of capers, rinsed and drained
1 or 2 pinches of crushed hot red pepper flakes or to taste
Salt and freshly ground pepper to taste
Freshly chopped basil for garnish (optional)
Pitted black olives for garnish (optional)

Place eggplant cubes in a bowl with salt and cover with water. Place heavy plate inside bowl to weight down cubes, submerging them in brine. Set aside for 1½–2 hours. Roast bell peppers under broiler in oven until skins turn black and are easy to remove. Peel off skins and cut peppers into long strips. Set aside. Heat ¼ cup of olive oil in a large skillet over medium-low heat, add onions and garlic, and cook until soft. Do not brown. Add roasted pepper to mixture. Drain eggplant cubes, and pat dry with paper towels. Add another ¼ cup olive oil to skillet, return to medium heat, and sauté eggplant cubes until golden brown (15 minutes). Add zucchini to skillet and cook, adding more olive oil if needed. When zucchini is cooked, add tomatoes, lowering heat slightly; stir in wine and simmer until wine is evaporated and mixture turns to a jam consistency (about 20 minutes). Stir in capers and hot pepper flakes, and combine all vegetables with tomato sauce. Use a slotted spoon to stir, but don't break up vegetables. Add salt and pepper to taste. Before serving, add basil and black olives if desired.

Approx. 221 calories per serving
2g protein, 21g total fat, 3g saturated fat, 0 trans fat,
9g carbohydrates, 0 cholesterol, 43mg sodium, 2g fiber

GARLICKY SWISS CHARD
(MAKES 6 SERVINGS OR 3 CUPS)

2 bunches Swiss chard (about 1½ pounds each), cleaned and trimmed
3 tablespoons extra-virgin olive oil
6 cloves fresh garlic, minced
½ cup low-sodium, fat-free chicken broth
¼ teaspoon hot cherry peppers, finely minced
½ teaspoon salt, or to taste
¼ teaspoon freshly ground pepper

Rinse greens well and cut ribs and stems into 2-inch pieces. Set aside. Break leaves into roughly 2-inch pieces. Heat oil in a large heavy-bottomed skillet; add garlic and sauté until golden brown, stirring constantly. Add chard ribs and stems, broth, and hot peppers, cook until almost tender. Add leaves in bunches, stirring to wilt. Stir in salt, pepper. Cook covered, until tender and liquid is evaporated, stirring often.

Approx. 83 calories per serving
2g protein, 7g total fat, 1g saturated fat, 0 trans fat,
4g carbohydrates, 0.1mg cholesterol, 222mg sodium, 1g fiber

LEMON GARLIC ASPARAGUS
(MAKES 4–6 SERVINGS)

3 tablespoons extra-virgin olive oil
2 pounds fresh asparagus, cleaned, with ends trimmed
1 clove fresh garlic, crushed
Salt and freshly ground pepper to taste
2 tablespoons sweet orange juice
¾ teaspoon grated lemon peel
1 cup shredded fresh Parmesan cheese

In a large non-stick skillet, heat oil over medium heat until hot. Add asparagus, garlic, and salt and pepper; turn several times to coat asparagus with oil. Cover skillet and cook for 6–7 minutes, or until asparagus is tender and lightly browned. Remove from heat. Sprinkle with orange juice and lemon peel. Transfer to serving platter and top with Parmesan shavings.

Approx. 134 calories per serving
8g protein, 11g total fat, 4g saturated fat, 0 trans fat,
3g carbohydrates, 11mg cholesterol, 228mg sodium, 1g fiber

FAVA BEANS WITH PESTO SAUCE
(MAKES 6 SERVINGS)

Spicy Garlicky Pesto Sauce (page 354)
3 (15-ounce) cans cooked fava beans, rinsed and drained
6 large lettuce leaves
1 small red onion, chopped
½ red bell pepper, diced
½ yellow pepper, diced
Salt and freshly ground pepper to taste
Tomato wedges for garnish

In a small bowl, mix pesto sauce with fava beans. Arrange lettuce on platter or on individual plates. Pile pesto bean mixture on top of lettuce. Scatter onion and diced peppers over bean mixture. Add salt and pepper to taste and garnish with tomato wedges.

This dish also makes a great quick lunch.

Approx. 240 calories per serving
12g protein, 3g total fat, 0.6g saturated fat, 0 trans fat,
40g carbohydrates, 0 cholesterol, 500mg sodium, 10g fiber

FETA AND MIXED BEANS
(MAKES 6–8 SERVINGS)

1 (16-ounce) can light red kidney beans
1 (16-ounce) can cannellini beans, rinsed and drained
1 (16-ounce) can chickpeas, rinsed and drained
3 ounces fresh feta cheese, crumbled
1 cup finely chopped red onion
3 tablespoons chopped fresh mint
1½ tablespoons non-caloric sweetener
2 cloves fresh garlic, finely chopped
¼ teaspoon salt, or to taste
¼ teaspoon freshly ground pepper
2 tablespoons + 1 teaspoon fresh squeezed lemon juice
1 tablespoon balsamic vinegar
1 teaspoon extra-virgin olive oil
4 cups mixed greens

Combine beans, cheese, onion, and mint; add sweetener and mix well. Add to bean mixture garlic, salt and pepper, lemon juice, vinegar, and olive oil. Toss again. Place 1 cup of greens on each plate; divide bean mixture into four servings and top each plate of greens with bean mixture and serve.

This dish also makes a great quick lunch.

Approx. 151 calories per serving
11g protein, 3g total fat, 2g saturated fat, 0 trans fat,
26g carbohydrates, 9mg cholesterol, 449mg sodium, 8g fiber

TUSCAN BRAISED FENNEL
(MAKES 4 SERVINGS)

2 medium fennel bulbs
4 tablespoons extra-virgin olive oil
2 cloves garlic, peeled and sliced
Salt and freshly ground pepper to taste
2 cups low-sodium vegetable broth
Garnish with grated Parmesan cheese

Wash and trim bulbs, then cut off tops and reserve for garnish. Pat bulbs dry and cut into quarters. Place pieces of fennel, flat side down, in a heavy skillet, together with oil, garlic, and seasonings. Cook over moderate heat, turning, until fennel pieces are browned. Add broth, bring to a boil, cover, and reduce heat to simmer. Cook another 30–40 minutes until fennel is tender and liquid is absorbed. Sprinkle with cheese and serve.

Approx. 174 calories per serving
2g protein, 14g total fat, 2g saturated fat, 0 trans fat,
8g carbohydrates, 0 cholesterol, 103mg sodium, 1g fiber

CHICKPEAS WITH COUSCOUS
(MAKES 4 SERVINGS)

1½ cups low-sodium, fat-free chicken broth
⅓ cup couscous, uncooked
1 (15-ounce) can chickpeas, rinsed and drained
1 medium tomato, chopped
10 medium pitted black olives, sliced
1 stalk celery, finely chopped
2 large scallions, green and white parts, sliced into 1-inch pieces
¼ cup black seedless raisins
½ teaspoon cumin
¼ cup non-fat plain yogurt
Chopped fresh parsley (optional)

Bring chicken broth to a boil, remove from heat, and add couscous. Cover and let stand until couscous is tender and liquid is absorbed. Fluff with a fork and transfer to a bowl. Add chickpeas, tomato, olives, celery, scallions, raisins, and cumin. Stir to mix well and garnish with 1 table-spoon of yogurt and parsley.

This dish also makes a great quick lunch.

Approx. 207 calories per serving
10g protein, 3g total fat, 0.3g saturated fat, 0 trans fat,
38g carbohydrates, 0.25mg cholesterol, 362mg sodium, 6g fiber

SPICY COUSCOUS
(MAKES 4–6 SERVINGS)

2¼ teaspoons extra-virgin olive oil

4 cloves fresh garlic, minced

1 small onion, coarsely chopped

3 cups low-sodium vegetable broth or low-sodium, fat-free chicken broth

6 ounces dry couscous

2 teaspoons of ground cayenne pepper to taste

1 teaspoon Harissa (page 352)—add more or less according to degree of
spiciness desired

Cilantro leaves, finely chopped, to taste

Salt and freshly ground pepper to taste

In a skillet, heat 1 teaspoon oil, add garlic and onion, and sauté until golden. In a saucepan, bring broth and remaining oil to a boil. Place couscous in oven-safe dish and pour hot broth and garlic mixture over couscous; stir to mix. Let stand for 10 minutes, until broth is absorbed. Add cayenne, Harissa, cilantro, and salt and pepper to taste as you fluff couscous between fingers to separate grains. Cover tightly to keep warm. Sprinkle a small amount of cayenne and cilantro on top just before serving.

Approx. 124 calories per serving
4g protein, 1g total fat, 1g saturated fat, 0 trans fat,
24g carbohydrates, 0 cholesterol, 47mg sodium, 1g fiber

SAUTÉED VEGETABLES WITH FRESH THYME
(MAKES 4 SERVINGS)

2 medium raw leeks
1 medium red bell pepper
2 medium celery stalks
2 (6–7 ounce) zucchini
1 medium eggplant
4 tablespoons extra-virgin olive oil
Salt and freshly ground pepper to taste
2 tablespoons minced fresh thyme
5 medium garlic cloves, minced
2 tablespoons minced fresh parsley

Clean sand from leeks. Cut 2-inch pieces of white and green parts of leek, flatten each piece, and cut into ⅓-inch slices. Separate slices. Cut pepper in half, deseed, and cut into 2-inch strips. Peel strings from celery and cut into 2-inch pieces. Cut zucchini in half and then into pieces roughly ¼ inch by ¼ inch. Peel eggplant and cut into pieces roughly 2 inches by ½-inch thick. In a large skillet, heat 2 tablespoons of olive oil; sauté eggplant over medium heat. Sprinkle with salt, tossing constantly until crispy tender. Remove eggplant from skillet and set aside on a paper towel–dressed platter, to absorb excess oil from eggplant; place platter in heated oven to keep eggplant warm. Heat additional tablespoon of oil in eggplant skillet, add leeks, and cook about 5 minutes, stirring often. Add red pepper, celery, salt, pepper, and thyme; continue cooking, tossing often, until vegetables are crispy tender. With a slotted spoon, transfer mixture to eggplant platter. Add zucchini and additional tablespoon of oil, if needed, to skillet, and cook zucchini until tender. Remove zucchini to eggplant platter. Add garlic to skillet and sauté for about 30 seconds; do not brown. Add parsley and heat an additional 2–3 seconds. Transfer all vegetables from eggplant platter to a clean platter. Pour garlic and parsley mixture over vegetables and toss, mixing well. Serve immediately.

Approx. 177 calories per serving
2g protein, 14g total fat, 2g saturated fat, 0 trans fat,
13g carbohydrates, 0 cholesterol, 22mg sodium, 2g fiber

CINNAMON COUSCOUS
(MAKES 6–8 SERVINGS)

3 cups warmed water
Pinch of salt
½ tablespoon extra-virgin olive oil
6 ounces dry couscous
2 tablespoons ground cinnamon
¼ cup black seedless raisins
¼ cup low-calorie baking sweetener
4 tablespoons Mazahar (orange blossom water)
Coarsely chopped walnuts for garnish

Bring water to a boil; add salt and oil. Place couscous in an oiled oven-safe dish, and pour liquid over couscous. Add 1 tablespoon cinnamon, raisins, sweetener, and orange blossom water; let stand for about 10 minutes or until liquid is absorbed. Fluff couscous with fingers to separate grains. When ready to serve, top couscous with remaining cinnamon and walnuts.

Approx. 87 calories per serving
3g protein, 1g total fat, 1g saturated fat, 0 trans fat,
19g carbohydrates, 0 cholesterol, 4mg sodium, 1g fiber

SWISS CHARD AND ARBORIO RICE
(MAKES 6 SERVINGS)

5 cups low-sodium, fat-free chicken broth
2½ tablespoons extra-virgin olive oil
1 medium onion, chopped
1 ¾ cups Arborio or other short-grain rice
1 bunch Swiss chard (about 10 leaves), spines cut to ¼-inch pieces, leaves
coarsely chopped
½ teaspoon dried rosemary, crumbled
½ cup dry white wine
Salt and freshly ground pepper to taste
½ cup freshly grated Parmesan cheese (reserve a small amount for garnish, if
desired)

Bring broth to a simmer, cover, set aside, and keep moderately hot. In a heavy-bottomed skillet, heat oil and sauté onions until translucent. Add rice, chard, and rosemary; stir until chard wilts. Add wine and simmer until liquid is absorbed. Add 4 ½ cups of broth and simmer until rice is tender and creamy, stirring often, then add remaining ½ cup of broth slowly as needed if mixture appears too dry, cooking about 20 minutes. Add salt and pepper and Parmesan cheese to taste. Serve immediately, garnished with a small amount of cheese if desired.

Approx. 371 calories per serving
12g protein, 10g total fat, 2g saturated fat, 0 trans fat,
56g carbohydrates, 7mg cholesterol, 306mg sodium, 1g fiber

BASIC RICE PILAF

(MAKES 6 SERVINGS)

3 cups low-sodium, fat-free chicken broth
2½ tablespoons extra-virgin olive oil
¼ cup chopped blanched almonds
¼ cup toasted pine nuts
1 medium onion, finely chopped
1½ cups long-grain rice
2 cups frozen peas
Salt and freshly ground pepper to taste
Chopped fresh cilantro for garnish

Heat chicken broth to a slow simmer. Place 2 tablespoons oil in a heavy-bottomed skillet, and gently sauté almonds and pine nuts—toast but do not burn. Remove nuts from heat with a slotted spoon and set aside. Add onions to oil, sauté, and cook until soft; do not brown. Add rice to oil and sauté over medium heat for 10–15 minutes, stirring constantly until rice is crispy. Pour in hot chicken broth, and add peas, ½ tablespoon olive oil, and salt and pepper to taste. Reduce heat, cover, and simmer until liquid is absorbed, about 20 minutes. Remove from heat, genrly fold in both nuts, cover, and set aside for 5 minutes before serving. Garnish with chopped cilantro.

Approx. 327 calories per serving
9g protein, 16g total fat, 2g saturated fat, 0 trans fat,
40g carbohydrates, 1mg cholesterol, 6mg sodium, 1g fiber

ROASTED GARLIC
(MAKES 4 SERVINGS)

1 jumbo garlic (4–5 large cloves)
Seasoned garlic salt to taste (optional)
Extra-virgin olive oil to drizzle

Cut the point off jumbo garlic cloves and remove loose leaves; try to keep cloves intact. Place in an oven-safe dish, sprinkle with a small amount of garlic salt, and drizzle with oil. Bake at 400 degrees for 20–30 minutes, or until cloves are soft and golden brown.

Great with crusty bread or pita wedges. Also great as a topper on cooked vegetables and omelets.

Approx. 59 calories per serving (based roughly on 4–5 servings per entire jumbo garlic)
3g protein, 0.2g total fat, <0.1g saturated fat, 0 trans fat,
13g carbohydrates, 0 cholesterol, 7mg sodium, 1g fiber

POLENTA
(MAKES 4–6 SERVINGS)

3 cups water
1 cup polenta
Extra-virgin olive oil (optional)
Grated Parmesan cheese for garnish (optional)
Salt and freshly ground pepper to taste

Bring water to boil in a saucepan. Slowly add polenta and bring back to a boil, stirring constantly. Lower heat to a simmer; stir frequently for roughly 20–25 minutes or until polenta thickens. Serve drizzled with olive oil and sprinkled with cheese. Add salt and freshly ground pepper to taste.

Approx. 35 calories per serving
1g protein, 4g total fat, 0 saturated fat, 0 trans fat,
6g carbohydrates, 0 cholesterol, 82mg sodium, 0 fiber

BAKED EGGPLANT WITH GARLIC AND BASIL
(MAKES 4–6 SERVINGS)

2 medium eggplants
Olive oil cooking spray
4 cloves fresh garlic, finely chopped
4 tablespoons extra-virgin olive oil
1½ teaspoons chopped fresh basil
1 tablespoon tomato paste
2 tablespoons freshly grated Parmesan cheese
Finely chopped fresh rosemary
Salt and freshly ground pepper to taste

Wash and dry eggplants, then cut each in half lengthwise. With a sharp knife, make a crisscross pattern in the skin of each eggplant. Put eggplants skin side down on a lightly oiled baking sheet and set aside. Mix together garlic, oil, basil, and tomato paste. Spread mixture onto tops of eggplants and bake at 350 degrees for 45 minutes or until tender. Remove from oven and garnish with cheese, rosemary, and salt and pepper to taste.

Approx. 97.6 calories per serving
1g protein, 10g total fat, 2g saturated fat, 0 trans fat,
3g carbohydrates, 1mg cholesterol, 51mg sodium, 1g fiber

POLENTA WITH MUSHROOMS AND GARLIC
(MAKES 4–6 SERVINGS)

1 tablespoon extra-virgin olive oil
3 large cloves garlic, minced
3 ounces white button mushroom, cleaned and sliced
2 sprigs thyme, stalks removed
3 cups water
1 cup polenta
Salt and freshly ground pepper to taste

In a skillet, heat oil and gently sauté garlic and mushrooms until soft. Add thyme, stir to blend, and set aside. Bring water to a boil, add polenta, and continue boiling for 2–3 minutes before reducing to a simmer. Cook, stirring frequently, for about 20–25 minutes, until polenta thickens and liquid is absorbed. Remove from heat, transfer to a bowl, stir in mushroom mixture, and add salt and pepper to taste.

Approx. 59 calories per serving
1g protein, 3g total fat, 0.3g saturated fat, 0 trans fat,
7g carbohydrates, 0 cholesterol, 83mg sodium, 0.2g fiber

GARLICKY CANNELLINI BEANS
(MAKES 4–6 SERVINGS)

2 (15-ounce) cans cannellini beans
4–5 large fresh cloves garlic, minced
2 tablespoons extra-virgin olive oil
½ cup low-sodium, fat-free chicken broth
Salt and freshly ground pepper to taste

Rinse and drain beans. Cook garlic and oil in a skillet over moderate heat until garlic softens, then add chicken broth and beans and simmer until most of the liquid is evaporated. Season with salt and pepper and serve with toasted pita.

Approx. 123 calories per serving
6g protein, 5g total fat, 0.6g saturated fat, 0 trans fat,
18g carbohydrates, 0.2mg cholesterol, 372mg sodium, 7g fiber

SAUTÉED PORTOBELLOS WITH GARLIC AND PARSLEY
(MAKES 4 SERVINGS)

2 tablespoons extra-virgin olive oil
12 ounces portobello mushrooms, cut into chunks
Salt and freshly ground pepper to taste
4 cloves fresh garlic, finely minced
1 tablespoon finely chopped parsley

In a skillet, heat oil and sauté mushrooms over high heat for about 4 minutes. Add salt and pepper to taste. Sprinkle with garlic and parsley and serve hot.

Approx. 81 calories per serving
2g protein, 7g total fat, 1g saturated fat, 0 trans fat,
4g carbohydrates, 0 cholesterol, 3mg sodium, 1g fiber

GRILLED EGGPLANT

(MAKES 4 SERVINGS)

1 tablespoon extra-virgin olive oil
2 tablespoons fresh oregano leaves
2 plum tomatoes, diced
1½ pounds eggplant, cut lengthwise into ½-inch thick slices
Olive oil cooking spray
2 large garlic cloves, finely minced
1 teaspoon chopped dried rosemary
Salt and freshly ground pepper to taste
¼ cup crumbled feta cheese
Lemon wedges
Oregano sprigs for garnish

Heat oil in saucepan, add oregano leaves, then remove pan from heat. Add tomato to oregano and allow to bathe in hot oil until ready to serve. Meanwhile, spray both sides of eggplant with olive oil spray, sprinkle with garlic, rosemary, and salt and pepper, and place on medium-hot grill. Cover grill and cook eggplant until tender and browned on both sides, turning once. Remove eggplant to platter, drizzle with oregano tomato oil, and top with feta cheese. Garnish with lemon wedges and oregano sprigs.

Approx. 74 calories per serving
4g protein, 6g total fat, 1g saturated fat, 0 trans fat,
10g carbohydrates, 5mg cholesterol, 86mg sodium, 0.2g fiber

GINGERED GREEN BEANS AND PEA PODS
(MAKES 4 SERVINGS)

8 ounces fresh green beans, washed and trimmed

2 cups low-sodium, fat-free chicken broth

2 teaspoons extra-virgin olive oil

2 cloves fresh garlic, finely chopped

½ teaspoon freshly ground ginger

4 ounces snow peas, washed, with strings removed (do not remove peas from pods)

4 ounces sugar peas, washed, with strings removed (do not remove peas from pods)

1 tablespoon low-sodium soy sauce

Freshly ground pepper to taste

In a large pan, steam green beans in chicken broth for about 3–4 minutes. Drain beans. In a clean skillet, add 1 teaspoon oil and green beans; sauté for about 2–3 minutes until they start to brown. Add remaining oil, garlic, ginger, snow peas, and sugar peas. Continue sautéing another 2–3 minutes, until pea pods are crispy tender. Stir in soy sauce and freshly ground pepper, and serve while hot.

Approx. 63 calories per serving

4g protein, 2g total fat, 0 saturated fat, 0 trans fat,

5g carbohydrates, 0 cholesterol, 187mg sodium, 3g fiber

STEAMED ARTICHOKES
(MAKES 4 SERVINGS)

4 medium globe artichokes (about 10–11 ounces each)
4 cups low-sodium, fat-free chicken broth
10 cloves fresh garlic
Salt and freshly ground pepper to taste
Extra-virgin olive oil or melted trans fat–free canola/olive oil spread to
drizzle (optional)

Wash artichokes under running water. Remove the sharp tips of each leaf with poultry scissors, keeping the globe intact. Place artichokes, broth, and garlic in a large pot. Cover pot and bring to a boil. Reduce heat to medium, keep pot covered, and continue to steam artichokes, turning over once while steaming. If necessary, add water to pot to keep artichokes bathed in liquid while steaming. Steam until you can pierce the globe stem area of the artichoke with a fork without much resistance. Remove chokes with a slotted spoon to serving dishes, sprinkle with salt and pepper, and drizzle with olive oil or melted canola/olive oil spread if desired. Serve while warm.

To eat this delectable vegetable, simply pull off the leaves one by one and run the soft flesh of the leaf over your bottom front teeth, extracting the flesh from the inner part of the leaf. In the center of all the leaves is the best part; the heart of the choke connected to the stem is also very good. The only part not considered edible by most people is the crown of fuzzy little leaves which sits directly on top of the heart. Simply remove these fuzzy little leaves with your fingers before eating the heart and stem.

Approx. 76 calories per serving
5g protein, 0.2g total fat, 0.1g saturated fat, 0 trans fat,
17g carbohydrates, 0 cholesterol, 153mg sodium, 5g fiber

MOM'S BROWN RICE
(MAKES 8 SERVINGS)

4 cups low-sodium, low-fat chicken broth
2 cups brown rice (uncooked)
6 cloves fresh garlic
½ cup pine nuts
6 scallions, white and green parts, trimmed and sliced
8 pitted large black olives, drained and coarsely chopped
½ tablespoon extra-virgin olive oil
Salt and freshly ground pepper to taste
Chopped chives for garnish

In a saucepan, bring broth and rice to a boil; reduce heat to medium, cover, and continue boiling until all liquid is absorbed, stirring occasionally if needed. While rice is boiling, sauté garlic, pine nuts, scallions, and olives in oil until garlic is soft and pine nuts are lightly toasted. When rice is ready, fluff with a fork and stir in garlic and pine nut mixture; add salt and pepper to taste. Transfer to serving platter and garnish with chopped chives.

Approx. 249 calories per serving
7g protein, 9g total fat, 1g saturated fat, 0 trans fat,
38g carbohydrates, 1mg cholesterol, 58mg sodium, 1g fiber

BAKED SWEET POTATO FRIES WITH BASIL PESTO
(MAKES 2 SERVINGS)

2 (6-ounce) sweet potatoes
1 tablespoon fresh Basil Pesto Sauce (page 357) or market-fresh basil pesto
Salt and freshly ground pepper to taste
Low-fat or fat-free sour cream, for garnish (optional)

Clean skins of sweet potatoes under cold running water and pat potatoes dry with paper towels. Cut potatoes in half and then each half into fry strips. Place fries in a single layer on a non-stick baking sheet and brush with pesto sauce. Add salt and pepper as desired. Place baking sheet in oven and bake fries at 400 degrees until tender and lightly browned around edges. Divide fries into two servings, and garnish with a dollop of sour cream.

Approx. 211 calories per serving
4g protein, 7g total fat, 1g saturated fat, 0 trans fat,
34g carbohydrates, 5mg cholesterol, 152mg sodium, 4g fiber

GREEN BEANS AND BABY PORTOBELLOS
(MAKES 4 SERVINGS)

12 ounces fresh green beans, ends snipped
1¼ cups sliced baby portobello mushrooms
1½ tablespoons finely chopped garlic
½ teaspoon onion powder
2 tablespoons trans fat–free canola/olive oil spread
Salt and freshly ground pepper to taste

In a medium saucepan add beans and mushrooms plus enough water to fill ⅓ of pan. Bring to a boil, then reduce heat and cook until beans are tender. Drain well and transfer beans and mushrooms to a large heavy-bottomed skillet. Add chopped garlic, onion powder, and canola/olive oil spread, and heat over low heat to melt, stirring often to coat beans and mushrooms. Continue to cook on low heat for at least 15 minutes to marry flavors. Add salt and pepper to taste if desired.

Approx. 74 calories per serving
2g protein, 5g total fat, 1g saturated fat, 0 trans fat,
7g carbohydrates, 0 cholesterol, 52mg sodium, 2g fiber

GARLIC ROASTED CAULIFLOWER
(MAKES 4 SERVINGS)

1 jumbo garlic clove, finely chopped
1 medium head of cauliflower (about 3 pounds), cut into 1½-inch florets
2 tablespoons extra-virgin olive oil
Garlic salt or seasoning of choice to taste (optional)

Place garlic, florets, and oil in a large Ziploc bag and toss to coat florets with oil and garlic. Arrange florets in a single layer in a shallow baking pan and sprinkle with seasoning if desired. Place pan on middle rack of 425-degree oven and roast cauliflower until tender and golden brown (about 20–30 minutes). Stir and turn florets over occasionally while roasting.

Approx. 91 calories per serving
3g protein, 7g total fat, 0.8g saturated fat, 0 trans fat,
7g carbohydrates, 0 cholesterol, 20mg sodium, 3g fiber

SAUTÉED GARLIC SPINACH
(MAKES 4 SERVINGS)

1½ cups low-sodium, fat-free chicken broth
4–6 fresh garlic cloves, chopped
3 (10-ounce) bags fresh spinach leaves
Freshly ground pepper to taste
Salt to taste

In a heavy-bottomed skillet over medium heat add chicken broth and garlic. Add handfuls of spinach while stirring, moving wilted leaves to one side, until all of the spinach has been added and wilted. Reduce heat to low, add pepper, and stir occasionally to blend garlic and spinach, until broth has evaporated. Add salt to taste. Serve while hot.

Approx. 54 calories per serving
5g protein, 0.2g total fat, 0 saturated fat, 0 trans fat,
7g carbohydrates, 2mg cholesterol, 174mg sodium, 4.5g fiber

GRILLED JUMBO PORTOBELLO MUSHROOMS
(MAKES 4 SERVINGS)

4 large (4–6-inch) portobello mushrooms
1 tablespoon balsamic vinegar
1 tablespoon Worcestershire sauce
⅓ cup extra-virgin olive oil
Freshly ground pepper to taste
Salt to taste

Wash and clean mushrooms. Mix marinade ingredients together, place mushrooms in a plastic Ziploc bag, and pour marinade over mushrooms. Seal bag and gently toss mushrooms and marinade to cover mushrooms. Refrigerate and marinate for 1–2 hours. Heat grill, place mushrooms on grill, and brush tops with remaining marinade. Grill each side for 5–6 minutes, or until mushrooms are soft. Turn mushrooms over once, brushing marinade mixture onto other side.

Approx. 98 calories per serving
0.6g protein, 9.8g total fat, 1g saturated fat, 0 trans fat,
2g carbohydrates, 0 cholesterol, 39mg sodium, 0.4g fiber

ARTICHOKE RISOTTO
(MAKES 4–6 SERVINGS)

1 (15-ounce) can quartered artichokes
2 tablespoons extra-virgin olive oil
1 small white onion, finely chopped
2 cloves garlic, finely chopped
1½ cups of short-grain rice
3 cups low-sodium, fat-free chicken broth
Salt and freshly ground pepper to taste
2 tablespoons parsley, finely chopped
¼ cup Parmesan cheese, freshly grated (optional)
Sprig of fresh parsley for garnish

Drain liquid from artichokes and set aside. Heat oil over medium heat; add onion and garlic, and sauté until soft. Add drained artichokes and cook another 5 minutes. Turn heat up to medium-high, add rice, and sauté another 2 minutes, stirring often to keep rice from burning. Add already-warmed chicken broth 1 cup at a time, stirring often and allowing rice to absorb most of the broth before adding the second and then third cup. Cook until rice is tender and broth is absorbed (about 15–20 minutes). Add salt and pepper to taste, and stir in parsley and cheese. Mix well and serve, garnished with a sprig of parsley.

Approx. 229 calories per serving
5g protein, 4g total fat, 0.3g saturated fat, 0 trans fat,
41 carbohydrates, 0 cholesterol, 124mg sodium, 3g fiber

Wraps and Sandwiches

ROASTED RED PEPPER SANDWICH
(MAKES 2 SERVINGS)

1 whole wheat pita loaf, split in half and toasted
2 pieces Roasted Peppers (page 237), or 2 pieces red bell peppers
1 ounce hard Parmesano-Reggiano cheese, sliced in thin pieces
½ cup alfalfa sprouts
4–6 Romaine lettuce leaves, broken
Salt and freshly ground pepper to taste
Garnish with a few black olives

Split pita loaf in half, open pocket of each side of loaf, and lightly toast. Insert 1 large piece of roasted pepper into each ½ pita pocket (the rest can be stored in the refrigerator in a sealed jar); add ½ of cheese to each pocket as well as sprouts, lettuce, and salt and pepper to taste. Serve garnished with black olives.

Approx. 145 calories per serving
8g protein, 3.6g total fat, 2.3g saturated fat, 0 trans fat,
11mg cholesterol, 215mg sodium, 3g fiber

LAMB WRAP
(MAKES 4 SERVINGS)

⅓ cup medium-grain bulgur
½ cup diced tomatoes
½ cup finely chopped fresh parsley
¼ cup finely chopped fresh mint leaves, no stems
2 scallions, thinly sliced
2 tablespoons extra-virgin olive oil
Juice from ½ lemon
Salt and freshly ground pepper to taste
½ tablespoon extra-virgin olive oil
2 cloves garlic, minced
½ pound lean ground lamb
4 ounces plain non-fat yogurt
¾ cup diced cucumbers
1 tablespoon chopped fresh mint
4 (6-inch) whole wheat pita loaves (do not split open)
1 cup chopped fresh spinach leaves
4 ounces crumbled fat-free feta cheese

Cover bulgur in a bowl with fresh cold water to a depth of roughly ½ inch. Let stand until water is absorbed (about 30 minutes). Fluff with a fork to separate grains. Grains should be plump and slightly moist; if too moist, spread grains on towel, fold towel, and squeeze to remove excess water. Combine tomatoes, parsley, mint, scallions, and olive oil. Add bulgur and toss gently. Squeeze lemon juice over tabbouleh mixture and refrigerate. Heat olive oil, and sauté garlic, lamb, and salt and pepper over medium-high heat until browned, stirring constantly to crumble. Drain well and set aside. Combine yogurt, cucumbers, and mint in small bowl, stir well, and set aside. Stack pita rounds and wrap in wax paper; microwave on high for 45 seconds. In a bowl, combine lamb mixture, spinach, and feta. Spoon ½ cup tabbouleh mixture and ¼ lamb mixture in the center of each pita round. Top with yogurt mixture and roll up pita. To secure, wrap bottom portion of pita roll-up with wax paper.

Approx. 462 calories per serving
21g protein, 22g total fat, 6g saturated fat, 0 trans fat,
43g carbohydrates, 43mg cholesterol, 635mg sodium, 5g fiber

VEGGIE WRAP
(MAKES 6 SERVINGS)

Olive oil cooking spray
2 medium tomatoes, cut into ½-inch thick slices
2 small cucumbers, sliced lengthwise into ½-inch thick slices
2 small onions, cut into ½-inch thick slices
1 green bell pepper, cut into strips
2 medium zucchini, sliced lengthwise into ½-inch thick slices
Extra-virgin olive oil to drizzle
¾ tablespoon crumbled dried oregano
¼ tablespoon crumbled dried rosemary
¾ teaspoon dried thyme
½ (7-ounce) can chickpeas, rinsed and drained
¼ teaspoon cumin (optional)
Salt and freshly ground pepper to taste
6 whole wheat flat bread (8–10-inch), warmed
Alfalfa sprouts (optional)

Spray non-stick pan with cooking spray. Place tomatoes, cucumbers, onions, peppers, and zucchini on pan, and drizzle with olive oil. Sprinkle with oregano, rosemary, and thyme, and roast for 15–20 minutes at 425 degrees. Add chickpeas and cumin, plus salt and pepper to taste, and cook an additional 15–20 minutes until tender. Fill warmed flat bread with bean and veggie mix, top with alfalfa sprouts, roll up, and serve.

Approx. 170 calories per serving
8g protein, 1g total fat, <0.3g saturated fat, 0 trans fat,
36g carbohydrates, 0 cholesterol, 325mg sodium, 6g fiber

CRAB AND AVOCADO STUFFED PITA POCKETS
(MAKES 8 SERVINGS)

⅔ cup light mayonnaise
4 tablespoons fresh lemon juice
2 tablespoons chopped Roasted Peppers (page 237)
Pinch cayenne pepper
1 pound (about 2 cups) lump crab meat, well drained
1 cup chopped pre-cooked shrimp
2 small avocados, chopped
3 tablespoons finely chopped white onion
Salt and freshly ground pepper to taste
4 whole grain pita loaves, cut in half
1 cup alfalfa sprouts

Blend together mayonnaise, lemon juice, roasted pepper, and cayenne, then refrigerate to chill (about 1 hour). Mix together crab, shrimp, avocados, onions, and salt and pepper to taste. Fill each pita loaf half with crab mixture and top with ⅛ of mayonnaise mixture. Add ⅛ cup of alfalfa sprouts to each filled pita and serve.

Approx. 171 calories per serving
11.6g protein, 12.4g total fat, 1.7g saturated fat, 0 trans fat,
4.6g carbohydrates, 61.5mg cholesterol, 216mg sodium, 1g fiber

GRILLED JUMBO PORTOBELLO MUSHROOM SANDWICH
(MAKES 4 SERVINGS)

4 large (4–6-inch) portobello mushrooms
1 tablespoon balsamic vinegar
1 tablespoon Worcestershire sauce
⅓ cup extra-virgin olive oil
Salt and freshly ground pepper to taste
1 whole grain hamburger bun
Condiments of choice (optional)

Wash and clean mushrooms. Mix together vinegar, Worcestershire sauce, olive oil, and salt and pepper, then place mushrooms in a plastic Ziploc bag and pour mixture over mushrooms. Seal bag and gently toss mushrooms and marinade to cover mushrooms. Refrigerate and marinate for 1–2 hours. Heat grill, place mushrooms on grill, and brush tops with remaining marinade. Grill each side for 5–6 minutes, or until mushrooms are soft. Turn mushrooms over once, brushing marinade mixture onto other side before grilling. Place on whole grain bun and add condiments of choice.

Approx. 248 calories per serving
5g protein, 11.8g total fat, 1.5g saturated fat, 0 trans fat,
29g carbohydrates, 0 cholesterol, 39mg sodium, 2.4g fiber

STUFFED WHOLE WHEAT KHUBZ
(MAKES 8 SERVINGS)

4 (6-inch) pita loaves
2 tablespoons stone-ground mustard
1 teaspoon finely chopped fresh cilantro
2 cloves garlic, finely crushed
⅛ teaspoon freshly ground pepper
Garlic salt to taste
1½ teaspoons extra-virgin olive oil
¼ teaspoon balsamic glaze
½ medium red onion, finely sliced
10 medium pitted black olives
1½ cups shredded lettuce
½ cup chopped carrot
½ cup diced celery
1 large tomato, diced
4 ounces crumbled feta cheese

Split pita loaves crosswise in half, spread open pockets (to keep from sealing shut), and lightly toast. Spread inside of toasted pockets with thin layer of mustard. Set aside. Mix cilantro, garlic, pepper, and garlic salt with olive oil and glaze, stir together to blend well, and then set aside. Combine onion, olives, lettuce, carrots, celery, and tomato, toss to mix, and fill pockets with vegetable blend. Drizzle each stuffed loaf with glaze mixture, and add crumbled feta. Serve.

Approx. 152 calories per serving
6g protein, 4g total fat, 2g saturated fat, 0 trans fat,
18g carbohydrates, 12mg cholesterol, 353mg sodium, 3g fiber

SPICY HUMMUS IN TOASTED PITA LOAVES
(MAKES 6 SERVINGS)

1 (15-ounce) can chickpeas, well rinsed and drained
Juice from 1 lemon
¼ cup water
1 large garlic clove
2 tablespoons tahini paste
Dash of salt
Pinch of red hot pepper flakes
3 (6-inch) whole wheat pita loaves, split in halves
8 slices tomatoes, ¼-inch thick
½ cucumber, peeled and thinly sliced
Alfalfa sprouts

In a food processor add chickpeas, lemon juice, and water, and blend to desired consistency. Add garlic, tahini paste, salt, and hot pepper flakes; blend again. Cut pita loaves in half, and toast lightly. Divide mixture into 4 portions and stuff loaves with mixture. Top each half loaf with tomato, cucumber, and alfalfa sprouts.

Approx. 152 calories per serving
3g protein, 3g total fat, 0.3g saturated fat, 0 trans fat,
27g carbohydrates, 0 cholesterol, 235mg sodium, 4g fiber

CHICKPEA PITA POCKETS
(MAKES 8 SERVINGS)

1 (15-ounce) can chickpeas, rinsed and drained
1 cup shredded fresh spinach
⅔ cup halved seedless red grapes
½ cup finely chopped red bell pepper
⅓ cup thinly sliced celery
½ medium cucumber, diced
¼ cup finely chopped onion
¼ cup light mayonnaise
1 tablespoon balsamic syrup
½ tablespoon poppy seed
4 (6-inch) whole wheat pita loaves, cut in half

In a large bowl combine chickpeas, spinach, grapes, red pepper, celery, cucumber, and onion. Whisk together mayonnaise, balsamic syrup, and poppy seeds. Add poppy seed mixture to chickpea mixture, and stir until well blended. Lightly toast pita halves and fill with chickpea filling. Serve.

Approx. 152 calories per serving
7g protein, 3g total fat, 0.3g saturated fat, 0 trans fat,
29g carbohydrates, 3mg cholesterol, 294mg sodium, 5g fiber

SPICY MUSHROOM WRAP
(MAKES 2 SERVINGS)

Olive oil cooking spray
1 tablespoon extra-virgin olive oil
2 large portobello mushrooms, sliced
2 teaspoons minced fresh garlic
½ small white onion, thinly sliced
2 teaspoons spicy brown mustard
½ pound arugula, trimmed and steamed
10 cherry tomatoes, halved
¼ cup shredded part-skim mozzarella cheese
2 light whole grain trans fat–free wraps
¼ hot cherry pepper, diced (optional)

Spray baking dish with cooking spray. In a large skillet, heat olive oil, and sauté mushrooms, garlic, and onion for about 5 minutes, stirring constantly. Put mustard, arugula, tomato, mozzarella, and cooked mushroom mixture on each tortilla. Sprinkle hot peppers down center if desired; roll up and place seam side down in oiled baking dish. Bake uncovered for 10 minutes or until cheese is melted. Serve.

Approx. 199 calories per serving
15g protein, 13g total fat, 2.5g saturated fat, 0 trans fat,
20g carbohydrates, 8mg cholesterol, 513mg sodium, 10mg fiber

CHICKPEA AND FRESH SPINACH SANDWICH
(MAKES 4 SERVINGS)

1 (15-ounce) can chickpeas
2 teaspoons extra-virgin olive oil
2 cloves fresh garlic, minced
½ medium white onion, diced
Salt and freshly ground pepper to taste
Red pepper flakes if desired
8 slices whole wheat grain bread
1 clove fresh garlic, cut in half
5–6 ounces fresh spinach leaves

Rinse and drain chickpeas thoroughly. Mash to a paste, and set aside. In 1 teaspoon olive oil, sauté minced garlic and diced onion until golden brown. Add chickpea paste and salt and pepper to taste, and red pepper flakes if desired. Drizzle paste with remaining teaspoon of oil and set aside. Toast whole wheat bread slices and rub one side of each piece with fresh garlic halves. Divide paste mixture and spinach leaves into 4 portions and make into 4 sandwiches. Serve.

Approx. 227 calories per serving
15g protein, 5g total fat, 0.3g saturated fat, 0 trans fat,
40g carbohydrates, 0 cholesterol, 600mg sodium, 11g fiber

SMOKED FISH AND ROASTED PEPPER SANDWICH
(MAKES 4 SERVINGS)

2 tablespoons extra-virgin olive oil
1 clove fresh garlic, mashed into a paste
8 slices whole wheat grain bread
3 ounces smoked white fish
3 ounces smoked sturgeon
4 tablespoons romaine lettuce
4 teaspoons diced Roasted Peppers (page 237)
2 teaspoons light mayonnaise

Combine oil and garlic, reserving 1 teaspoon. Lightly brush both sides of bread with mixture and toast in oven at 350 degrees for 4 minutes, or until golden brown. Set aside. Mix fish, lettuce, and roasted peppers together; set aside. Blend mayonnaise and 1 teaspoon oil together, and add to fish mixture. Divide mixture into 4 servings and spread onto bread, making 4 sandwiches.

Approx. 228 calories per serving
19g protein, 11g total fat, 1g saturated fat, 0 trans fat,
20g carbohydrates, 8mg cholesterol, 463mg sodium, 4g fiber

Breads

Wheat flour is the most common variety of flour used for making bread. However, other types such as barley flour, bran, buckwheat flour, cornmeal, rolled oats, oat flour, and soy flour—to mention just a few—are also suitable for bread making. All flours should be stored in airtight containers. All-purpose and white bread flour can be stored at 70 degrees for up to six months. Any flour, wheat or otherwise, which contains the germ from the grain can easily turn rancid. These flours should be stored in the refrigerator or freezer and can be kept for up to three months.

Homemade Breads

FOCACCIA
(MAKES 12 SQUARES)

A popular Italian bread found all over Italy. Usually round or rectangular in shape and about ½–1 inch thick. A variety of different toppings are used, such as herbs, coarse salt, a sprinkling of rosemary with hot pepper, olives, or even an array of vegetables.

1¼ cups hot water
1 package rapid-rising active dry yeast
3 tablespoons toasted wheat germ
1 tablespoon extra-virgin olive oil
Pinch of salt
2 cups durum whole wheat flour plus extra for kneading
Olive oil for brushing surfaces

Pour water into a medium-sized bowl and sprinkle with yeast. Stir with a wire whisk. Add wheat germ, olive oil, and pinch of salt, and whisk again. Add flour, then stir with a wooden spoon until dough forms a ball and leaves sides of bowl. Knead briefly, adding extra flour if needed, until dough is no longer sticky but still soft (about 3 minutes). Turn dough out onto a lightly floured surface; roll out into a rectangle, 11 inches by 17 inches. Lightly dust top with flour while rolling to prevent sticking. Ease dough into a lightly oiled 11x17-inch baking pan, stretch to fit, and cover with sheet of lightly oiled waxed paper, oiled side down. Allow to rise in a warm place for 25 minutes. After dough has risen, press dough with index finger to create little dimples over the surface. Add favorite topping and bake in 450-degree oven until lightly browned on the bottom (about 20–25 minutes). Remove and cool on rack. Slice into 12 large squares and serve.

Approx. 111 calories per square
4g protein, 1g total fat, <0.5g saturated fat, 0 trans fat,
23g carbohydrates, 0 cholesterol, 239mg sodium, 1g fiber

EGYPTIAN KHUBZ (PITA BREAD)
(MAKES 12 LOAVES)

The Arabs eat bread with every meal. They use it to scoop up sauces, dips, yogurt, and liquids. Pita cut in half can be filled with shish kabobs, falafel, or salads. They consider bread to be a divine gift from God.

1 package dried yeast
¼ teaspoon honey
1½ cups warm water
4 cups durum whole wheat flour
Pinch of salt
½ tablespoon extra-virgin olive oil
Cornmeal to dust baking sheet

Dissolve yeast and honey in 1 cup warm water and set aside for 5 minutes. Mix flour, salt, and oil in a large bowl, add yeast mixture and remaining water and mix well. Knead for 10 minutes until dough is elastic; then place dough in a warm, oiled bowl, cover with a dry cloth and set in a warm place to double its volume (about 2–3 hours). Punch dough down and knead again for about 2 more minutes. Form dough into 12 smooth balls the size of oranges. Place balls on a dry cloth in a warm place and cover to rise for another 30 minutes. Preheat oven to 500 degrees and lightly flour a board with cornmeal and roll out balls into ¼-inch thick circles. Bake loaves 5–8 minutes on a preheated baking sheet on center rack of oven. The loaves will puff up while baking but will collapse when cooled.

Approx. 218 calories per loaf
7g protein, 5g total fat, 0.5g saturated fat, 0 trans fat,
41g carbohydrates, 0 cholesterol, 497mg sodium, 10g fiber

LAVOSH

Same recipe as for pita bread, except pita bread is left in oven until it is golden brown and crisp. Once cooled, break bread into pieces.

Approx. 218 calories per loaf
7g protein, 5g total fat, 0.5g saturated fat, 0 trans fat,
41g carbohydrates, 0 cholesterol, 497mg sodium, 10g fiber

SESAME BREAD (KERSA)

(MAKES 2 16-INCH ROUND LOAVES; 12 SLICES/LOAF)

Kersa is a round, flat Moroccan bread that is slightly crunchy on the outside and chewy on the inside, great for dipping in soup or with stews.

1 package of active dry yeast
¼ cup + 2 cups warm water
1 teaspoon low-calorie baking sweetener
4 cups durum whole wheat semolina flour
2 teaspoons salt
⅓ cup cornmeal and extra for dusting
½ tablespoon extra-virgin olive oil
2 teaspoons sesame seeds

Using a small bowl, combine yeast with ¼ cup water, add sweetener, and let set until mixture starts to bubble. In a heavy-duty mixer bowl with dough hook mix flour, salt, and cornmeal. Indent center of dough, pour in yeast mixture and olive oil. Knead dough, adding remaining water as needed until dough takes on an elastic quality. Grease 2 baking sheets and dust with cornmeal. Separate dough to form 2 round balls and place each ball on a separate baking sheet. Press them into 8-inch circles. Sprinkle 1 teaspoon of sesame seeds over each loaf, gently pressing them into surface of dough. Cover dough with a clean cloth and set aside in a warm place for about 1 hour until they double their size. Preheat oven to 425 degrees. Prick the top of loaves with a fork and bake for 10 minutes. Lower heat to 375 degrees and bake loaves until top is crusty and golden brown, about 15–20 minutes.

Approx. 84 calories per slice
3g protein, 2g total fat, <0.5g saturated fat, 0 trans fat,
16g carbohydrates, 0 cholesterol, 90mg sodium, 1g fiber

Bread-Machine Breads

HONEY WHOLE WHEAT BREAD
(MAKES 20–22 SLICES)

⅔ cup + 3 tablespoons water
2 tablespoons canola oil
1½ teaspoons sodium-free salt substitute
1 tablespoon low-calorie brown sugar blend
2 tablespoons natural fat-free dry milk
2 tablespoons pure honey
2¾ cups whole wheat flour
2¼ teaspoons active dry yeast (at room temperature)

Remove baking machine canister. First, add water, then oil, salt substitute, sweetener, milk, and honey. Cover these ingredients with flour and finally yeast. Do not allow yeast to touch liquids. Return canister to machine per machine instructions, close lid, and follow setting instructions for making whole wheat bread. When machine is finished, remove loaf and allow to thoroughly cool before slicing. Store any unused bread in freezer.

Approx. 73 calories per slice
2g protein, 1g total fat, 0 saturated fat, 0 trans fat,
13g carbohydrates, 0 cholesterol, 2g sodium, 2g fiber

CRANBERRY NUT WHOLE WHEAT BREAD

(MAKES 20–22 SLICES)

¾ cup + 7 tablespoons water
2 tablespoons canola oil
1½ teaspoon sodium-free salt substitute
2 tablespoons low-calorie brown sugar blend
2 tablespoons natural fat-free dry milk
2¾ cups whole wheat flour
½ cup chopped dried cranberries
¼ cup sliced raw almonds
2¼ teaspoons active dry yeast (at room temperature)

Remove baking machine canister. First, add water, then oil, salt substitute, sweetener, and milk. Cover liquid ingredients with flour, cranberries, nuts, and finally yeast. Do not allow yeast to touch liquids. Return canister to machine per machine instructions, close lid, and follow setting instructions for making whole wheat bread. When machine is finished, remove loaf and allow to thoroughly cool before slicing. Store any unused bread in freezer.

Approx. 93 calories per slice
4g protein, 2g total fat, 0 saturated fat, 0 trans fat,
14g carbohydrates, 0 cholesterol, 1mg sodium, 3g fiber

MIXED FRUIT AND NUT WHOLE WHEAT BREAD
(MAKES 20–22 SLICES)

1¼ cups of water
2 tablespoons canola oil
1½ teaspoons sodium-free salt substitute
2 tablespoons low-calorie brown sugar blend
2 tablespoons natural fat-free dry milk
2¾ cups whole wheat flour
⅓ cup lightly salted pumpkin seeds
5 dried apricots, finely chopped
¼ cup white raisins
¼ cup sliced raw almonds
2¼ teaspoons active dry yeast (at room temperature)

Remove baking machine canister. First, add water, then oil, salt sub-stitute, sweetener, and milk. Cover these ingredients with flour, seeds, apricots, raisins, almonds, and finally yeast. Do not allow yeast to touch liquids. Return canister to machine per machine instructions, close lid, and follow setting instructions for making whole wheat bread. When machine is finished, remove loaf and allow to thoroughly cool before slicing. Store any unused bread in freezer.

Approx. 88 calories per slice
3g protein, 2g total fat, 1g saturated fat, 0 trans fat,
14g carbohydrates, 0 cholesterol, 3mg sodium, 2g fiber

NUTTY POMEGRANTE WHOLE WHEAT BREAD
(MAKES 20–22 SLICES)

1¼ cups of water

2 tablespoons canola oil

1½ teaspoons sodium-free salt substitute

2 tablespoons low-calorie brown sugar blend

2 tablespoons natural dry milk

2¾ cups whole wheat flour

Seeds from 1 pomegranate fruit

⅓ cup lightly salted pumpkin seeds

¼ cup sliced raw almonds

1½ teaspoons dried orange peel

2¼ teaspoons active dry yeast (at room temperature)

Remove baking machine canister. First, add water, then oil, salt substitute, sweetener, and milk. Cover these ingredients with flour, pomegranate and pumpkin seeds, almonds, orange peel, and finally yeast. Do not allow yeast to touch liquids. Return canister to machine per machine instructions, close lid, and follow setting instructions for making whole wheat bread. When machine is finished, remove loaf and allow to thoroughly cool before slicing. Store any unused bread in freezer.

Approx. 73 calories per slice
3g protein, 2g total fat, 0.1g saturated fat, 0 trans fat,
13g carbohydrates, 0 cholesterol, 2mg sodium, 2g fiber

NUTTY WHOLE WHEAT BREAD
(MAKES 20–22 SLICES)

1¼ cups of water
2 tablespoons canola oil
1½ teaspoons sodium-free salt substitute
2 tablespoons low-calorie brown sugar blend
2 tablespoons natural fat-free dry milk
2¾ cups whole wheat flour
¼ cup finely chopped raw walnuts
1½ teaspoons dried orange peel
⅓ cup lightly salted pumpkin seeds
2¼ teaspoons active dry yeast (at room temperature)

Remove baking machine canister. First, add water, then oil, salt substitute, sweetener, and milk. Cover these ingredients with flour, nuts, orange peel, seeds, and finally yeast. Do not allow yeast to touch liquids. Return canister to machine per machine instructions, close lid, and follow setting instructions for making whole wheat bread. When machine is finished, remove loaf and allow to thoroughly cool before slicing. Store any unused bread in freezer.

Approx. 79 calories per slice
3g protein, 2g total fat, 0.2g saturated fat, 0 trans fat,
12g carbohydrates, 0 cholesterol, 2mg sodium, 2g fiber

SUNDRIED TOMATO BASIL WHITE WHEAT BREAD
(MAKES 20–22 SLICES)

1½ cups water (room temperature)
2 tablespoons olive oil
2 teaspoons sodium-free salt substitute
3 tablespoons low-calorie brown sugar blend
3 tablespoons natural fat-free dry milk
3 tablespoons fresh sundried tomato pesto
8 large pitted black olives, chopped
10 sundried tomatoes, chopped
2 cups white wheat flour
2 cups bread flour
2 teaspoons active dry yeast

Remove baking machine canister. First, add water, then oil, salt substitute, sweetener, milk, pesto, olives, and sundried tomatoes. Cover these ingredients with flours, and finally yeast. Do not allow yeast to touch liquids. Return canister to machine per machine instructions, close lid, and follow setting instructions for making white wheat bread. When machine is finished, remove loaf and allow to thoroughly cool before slicing. Store any unused bread in freezer.

Approx. 104 calories per slice
4g protein, 11g total fat, 0.1g saturated fat, 0 trans fat,
14g carbohydrate, 0 cholesterol, 21mg sodium, 2g fiber

Desserts

FRESH FRUIT AND NUT PLATTER

A platter of seasonal fresh fruits and various types of nuts is often served alone or in mixed company at the end of a Mediterranean meal.

Great fruits to try include bananas, kiwi, figs, dates, strawberries, grapes, peaches, plums, pears, melons, apples, pomegranates, currants, and mandarin oranges.

STRAWBERRY AND POACHED PEARS
(MAKES 4 SERVINGS)

4 large ripe Anjou or Bartlett pears, peeled and cored
2 tablespoons fresh lemon juice
½ cup red wine (not cooking wine)
1½ cups water
2 tablespoons low-calorie baking sweetener
1 cinnamon stick
1 teaspoon freshly grated orange rind
½ teaspoon freshly grated lemon rind
¼ teaspoon cloves, ground
Fresh mint leaves for garnish

For Strawberry Sauce:

1 pint of fresh strawberries, cleaned and sliced
3 tablespoons non-caloric sweetener
1 teaspoon Grand Marnier liqueur

Slice off bottom of pears to allow them to sit flat in a pan. Brush body of pears with lemon juice. In a saucepan combine wine, water, sweetener, cinnamon, orange rind, lemon rind, and cloves. Bring to a boil over medium heat, reduce heat, and simmer for 5 minutes. Add pears, cover, and poach for 20 minutes until tender. Let pears stand in liquid until cool. Refrigerate until ready to serve. When serving, place pears on dessert plates and drizzle with a small amount of strawberry sauce. Garnish with mint leaf.

Strawberry Sauce:

Put strawberries in bowl and sprinkle with sweetener and Grand Marnier. Let stand at room temperature for 1 hour. Blend or process until puréed, then refrigerate sauce to chill.

Approx. 120 calories per serving
1g protein, 1g total fat, 0 saturated fat, 0 trans fat,
3g carbohydrates, 0 cholesterol, 2mg sodium, 4g fiber

FIGS IN PLAIN YOGURT
(MAKES 4 SERVINGS)

16 small figs
1½ cups red wine
2 tablespoons honey
¼ teaspoon ground cinnamon
2 cups plain low-fat yogurt
Non-caloric sweetener as desired
Finely chopped fresh mint for garnish

Slice open skins of figs on one side. Combine wine, honey, and cinnamon in a large saucepan and bring mixture to boil. Reduce to simmer, add figs, and simmer for 10–15 minutes. Remove from heat and allow figs to bathe in liquid for 5–10 minutes. Remove skins from figs and mash insides. Combine mashed figs with yogurt and mix well; add sweetener if desired. Refrigerate until well chilled. Divide yogurt mixture into 4 dessert bowls. Sprinkle with fresh mint.

Approx. 280 calories per serving
0.5g protein, 2g total fat, 1g saturated fat, 0 trans fat,
48g carbohydrates, 8mg cholesterol, 75mg sodium, 4g fiber

HONEY MOUSSE DELIGHT
(makes 6 servings)

⅓ cup honey
2 teaspoons freshly grated orange rind
12 ounces part skim-milk ricotta cheese
2½ cups halved fresh strawberries
2½ cups blackberries
¼ cup fresh orange juice
3 tablespoons non-caloric sweetener
2 tablespoons finely chopped walnuts

Mix honey, rind, and ricotta cheese in a medium bowl; cover, and re-frigerate to chill. Combine berries, juice, and sweetener, gently toss, and let stand for 5 minutes before covering and re-chilling. When well chilled, spoon ⅓ berry mixture (divided equally) into 6 serving bowls and top each with about ¼ cup of ricotta mixture. Divide remaining fruit mixture into 6 portions and add on top of cheese. Sprinkle with nuts and serve.

Approx. 196 calories per serving
7g protein, 6g total fat, 3g saturated fat, 0 trans fat,
29g carbohydrates, 18mg cholesterol, 71mg sodium, 1g fiber

SPICE CAKE
(MAKES 9 [1-INCH WIDE] SERVINGS)

½ teaspoon anise seed
¾ cup water
½ cup honey
½ cup low-calorie baking sweetener
½ teaspoon baking soda
3 cups unbleached white flour
⅛ teaspoon cinnamon
¼ teaspoon fresh grated nutmeg
Pinch of salt
⅛ cup mixed chopped orange and lemon peels
Olive oil cooking spray

In a medium saucepan bring anise seed covered with water to a boil; add honey and sweetener, and stir until both are dissolved. Remove mixture from heat and add baking soda. Sift flour, spices, and salt into a large bowl. Add orange and lemon peels. Strain liquid from anise seeds and mix into dry ingredients, stirring constantly. Beat until mixture is smooth, then pour into 9x5x3-inch sprayed and floured baking pan. Bake for 1 hour in a 350-degree oven, or until cake just begins to shrink from sides of pan. Remove from oven and let cool slightly. Serve warm or cool.

Approx. 360 calories per serving
8g protein, 0.7g total fat, 0.1g saturated fat, 0 trans fat,
83g carbohydrates, 0 cholesterol, 83mg sodium, 2g fiber

PEACH MARSALA COMPOTE
(MAKES 6 SERVINGS)

Canola oil cooking spray
12 fresh peaches
6 cups water
¾ cup low-calorie baking sweetener
½ cup Marsala wine
½ teaspoon ground cinnamon
½ teaspoon vanilla extract
½ teaspoon freshly grated nutmeg

Lightly spray a 2-quart baking dish with cooking spray. Blanch the peaches in boiling water for 20 seconds, then remove skin while holding under cold running water. Pit and slice peaches. Add peaches, sweetener, wine, cinnamon, vanilla extract, and nutmeg to a baking dish and bake for 45 minutes to 1 hour in a 350-degree oven. Serve warm or at room temperature.

Approx. 80 calories per serving
1g protein, 0.2g total fat, 0 saturated fat, 0 trans fat,
21g carbohydrates, 0 cholesterol, 126mg sodium, 3g fiber

SWEET PLUM COMPOTE
(MAKES 6 SERVINGS)

Canola oil cooking spray
3 pounds ripe plums, halved and pitted
¼ cup low-calorie baking sweetener
1 cup water
1 tablespoon Crème de Cassis liqueur

Lightly spray a baking dish with cooking spray. Add plums to baking dish. Combine sweetener and water in a saucepan and bring to a boil; cook for about 5 minutes, stirring constantly, or until liquid becomes syrupy. Pour syrup over plums and drizzle with Crème de Cassis. Bake mixture for 45 minutes to 1 hour in a 350-degree oven. Serve warm or cool.

Approx. 130 calories per serving
2g protein, 1g total fat, 0.1g saturated fat, 0 trans fat,
28g carbohydrates, 0 cholesterol, 1mg sodium, 1g fiber

SWEET MANGO MOUSSE
(MAKES 6 SERVINGS)

1¼ cups water
1 cup couscous
4 tablespoons non-caloric sweetener
¾ cup fresh orange juice
2 tablespoons orange-flavored liqueur
1 large ripe mango
1 cup light whipping cream, well chilled
1¼ teaspoons vanilla extract
1 (8-ounce) container low-fat vanilla yogurt
Orange zest, finely minced, for garnish

Bring water to a boil over medium-high heat. Add couscous slowly, stirring once, and remove from heat. Cover and set aside for 12–15 minutes, until couscous is tender. Add 2 tablespoons of sweetener, and mix well into couscous. Cover and set aside. In a small saucepan over medium heat, heat orange juice, stirring constantly until reduced to the consistency of honey (about 4–5 minutes). Stir in liqueur. Set aside. Peel the mango; cut half of flesh into thin wedges; coarsely dice the other half and set aside. Pour cream into a chilled bowl and whip until it peaks. Fold in vanilla and remaining sweetener. Divide in half, and set half aside. In a clean bowl combine remaining half of whipped cream, yogurt, and diced mango, and refrigerate until well chilled. Before serving, combine mango mixture with couscous. Divide into 6 equal portions, and top each portion with a good dollop of the remaining whipped cream and mango wedges. Drizzle with liqueur sauce, sprinkle with minced orange zest, and serve.

Approx. 316 calories per serving
7g protein, 19g total fat, 7.8g saturated fat, 0 trans fat,
40g carbohydrates, 46mg cholesterol, 44mg sodium, <1g fiber

FRESH FRUIT KABOBS AND CINNAMON HONEY DIP
(MAKES 2 SERVINGS)

*Assorted bite-sized chunks of your favorite fresh fruits (enough for 2 [8-inch]
wooden skewers)*
1 cup of low-fat plain yogurt
2 tablespoons of honey or non-caloric sweetener
Pinch of ground white pepper
6 teaspoons of ground cinnamon or to taste

Prepare fruits on skewers and set aside. Combine yogurt, honey, and white pepper, and mix well. Divide mixture into 2 individual serving bowls; sprinkle cinnamon on top of each serving and gently swirl in. Cover and refrigerate to chill before serving.

NOTE: Values shown are for yogurt dip only (values for fruit cannot be calculated since they depend on the specific fruits chosen).

Approx. 70 calories per serving
0.5g protein, 2g total fat, 1g saturated fat, 0 trans fat,
8g carbohydrates, 7mg cholesterol, 75mg sodium, 0 fiber

FRESH FRUIT IN YOGURT WITH RUM
(MAKES 2 SERVINGS)

¼ cup each of two of the following: blueberries, sliced strawberries, grapes,
   kiwi, or raspberries
2 cups low-fat plain yogurt
Dark rum (or other favorite liqueur) to taste
Non-caloric sweetener to taste (optional)

Cut up enough desired fresh fruit for 2 servings; add 2 cups plain yogurt and mix well. Divide mixture into two individual glass dessert cups and generously splash each serving with dark rum. Add sweetener if desired; chill before serving.

NOTE: Values shown are for yogurt dip only (values for fruit cannot be calculated since they depend on the specific fruits chosen).

Approx. 140 calories per serving
1g protein, 3.5g total fat, 2g saturated fat, 0 trans fat,
16g carbohydrates, 15mg cholesterol, 150mg sodium, 0 fiber

STUFFED DATES
(MAKES 16 DATES)

16 pitted dates
16 whole almonds
6 tablespoons almond paste

Slice dates open on one side. Pull back skin from the meat of the date and stuff each date with 1 almond and 1 teaspoon almond paste. Serve.

Approx. 152 calories per date
9g protein, 14g total fat, 1.2g saturated fat, 0 trans fat,
9g carbohydrates, 0 cholesterol, 0.8mg sodium, 3g fiber

SWEET ITALIAN RICE PUDDING
(MAKES 6 SERVINGS)

24 ounces evaporated skim milk
¼ cup long-grain rice
3 tablespoons low-calorie baking sweetener
1 teaspoon vanilla extract
Ground cinnamon

Combine 12 ounces milk and rice in a double boiler over water. Simmer, stirring frequently, for about 20 minutes. Add remaining milk and sweetener, and mix well. Return to a simmer, stirring often, until the mixture gains a pudding consistency (about 45 minutes). Add 1 teaspoon vanilla extract and blend into pudding while simmering for an additional few minutes. Remove from heat and sprinkle generously with cinnamon. Cool to room temperature, cover, and refrigerate before serving.

Approx. 117 calories per serving
9g protein, 0.5g total fat, 0.4g saturated fat, 0 trans fat,
19g carbohydrates, 4mg cholesterol, 133mg sodium, <0.5g fiber

CRÈME DE BANANA BAKED APPLES
(MAKES 4–6 SERVINGS)

4 medium sweet apples, peeled, cored, and halved
6 ounces unsweetened apple juice
2 teaspoons ground cinnamon
3 tablespoons pure honey
1 teaspoon vanilla extract
4 tablespoons Crème de Banana liqueur
1 cup plain fat-free yogurt
Non-caloric sweetener to taste

Place apples cored side up in a snugly fitting shallow baking dish. Add apple juice to just barely cover bottom halves of apples. Sprinkle with 1 teaspoon cinnamon, cover, and bake for 30–40 minutes in a 350-degree oven, or until apples are almost tender. Remove from oven and pour off any additional liquid, leaving just enough to cover bottom of dish. Drizzle tops of apples with honey, vanilla extract, liqueur, and remaining teaspoon of cinnamon. Bake for an additional 10 minutes. Remove from oven and divide equally onto 4 dessert plates. Blend yogurt and sweetener together and serve on the side.

Approx. 130 calories per serving
<.05g protein, <0.5g total fat, <.05g saturated fat, 0 trans fat,
27g carbohydrates, <1mg cholesterol, 28mg sodium, 2g fiber

CANTALOUPE SORBET
(MAKES 4–6 SERVINGS)

1½ cups of water
½ cup low-calorie baking sweetener
2 ripe cantaloupes, peeled, halved, seeded, and chunked
¼ cup fresh lemon juice
¼ cup egg whites
Mint sprigs for garnish

Combine water and sweetener, and bring to a boil over medium heat. Reduce heat and simmer for 5 minutes, then allow to cool. In a food processor or blender add cantaloupe and its juices, lemon juice, and cooled syrup. Puree until smooth. Pour mixture into bowl and freeze until almost frozen. Remove from freezer and beat with an electric beater until mixture is again smooth. Beat egg whites until stiff and fold into frozen fruit mixture. Cover container and freeze again until firm (about 2–3 hours). When ready to serve, scoop into dessert cups and garnish with mint sprigs if desired.

Approx. 67 calories per serving
2g protein, <0.5 total fat, 0 saturated fat, 0 trans fat,
15g carbohydrates, 0 cholesterol, 28mg sodium, 1g fiber

HONEYDEW SORBET
(MAKES 4–6 SERVINGS)

1½ cups of water
½ cup low-calorie baking sweetener
2 ripe honeydews (about 5 inches in diameter each), peeled, seeded, and
    chunked
¼ cup fresh lemon juice
¼ cup egg whites
Mint sprigs for garnish

Combine water and sweetener, and bring to a boil over medium heat. Reduce heat and simmer for 5 minutes, then allow to cool. In a food processor or blender add honeydew and its juices, lemon juice, and cooled syrup. Puree until smooth. Pour mixture into bowl and freeze until almost frozen. Remove from freezer and beat with an electric beater until mixture is again smooth. Beat egg whites until stiff and fold into frozen fruit mixture. Cover container and freeze again until firm (about 2–3 hours). When ready to serve, scoop into dessert cups and garnish with mint sprigs if desired.

Approx. 117 calories per serving
2g protein, <0.5g total fat, 0 saturated fat, 0 trans fat,
31g carbohydrates, 0 cholesterol, 33mg sodium, 2g fiber

STRAWBERRIES AND BALSAMIC SYRUP
(MAKES 4 SERVINGS)

2½ cups strawberries, hulled and halved
4 tablespoons Crème de Banana liqueur
Non-caloric sweetener to taste
Balsamic syrup

Combine strawberries and liqueur in a large bowl, toss well, cover, and refrigerate 20–30 minutes. When ready to serve, remove strawberries with a slotted spoon and place in a single layer on a dessert platter. Dust generously with sweetener, drizzle with balsamic syrup, and serve.

Approx. 49 calories per serving
<1g protein, 0.4g total fat, <0.1g saturated fat, 0 trans fat,
7g carbohydrates, 0 cholesterol, 1mg sodium, 2g fiber

DRUNKEN PEACHES
(MAKES 4 SERVINGS)

4 peaches
1½ cups red wine
1⅓ cups water
3 strips lemon peel (yellow part only)
3 tablespoons honey
1 cinnamon stick
Sprinkle with non-caloric sweetener to taste (optional)
Fat-free whipped cream (optional)

Peel skin from peaches. In a saucepan add wine, water, lemon peel, honey, and cinnamon stick, and bring to boil. Add peaches to sauce, submerging under liquid as much as possible, and gently poach for 5–10 minutes, until just tender. Remove peaches from saucepan and place in a bowl; set aside. Boil liquid in the saucepan, stirring constantly, until it becomes thick and syrupy. Remove cinnamon stick and lemon peel before liquid becomes dark. Pour syrup, when cool, over peaches, and serve. Garnish with sweetener and whipped cream if desired.

Approx. 115 calories per serving
1g protein, <.08g total fat, 0 saturated fat, 0 trans fat,
22g carbohydrates, 0 cholesterol, 0.5mg sodium, 1g fiber

DRUNKEN APRICOTS
(MAKES 4 SERVINGS)

8 medium apricots
1½ cups red wine
1⅓ cups water
3 strips lemon peel (yellow part only)
3 tablespoons honey
1 cinnamon stick
Sprinkle with non-caloric sweetener to taste (optional)
Fat-free whipped cream (optional)

Peel skin from apricots. In a saucepan add wine, water, lemon peel, honey, and cinnamon stick, and bring to boil. Add apricots to sauce, submerging under liquid as much as possible, and gently poach for 5–10 minutes, until just tender. Remove apricots from saucepan and place in a bowl; set aside. Boil liquid in the saucepan, stirring constantly, until it becomes thick and syrupy. Remove cinnamon stick and lemon peel before liquid becomes dark. Pour syrup, when cool, over apricots, and serve. Garnish with sweetener and whipped cream if desired.

Approx. 112 calories per serving
1g protein, 0.3g total fat, 0 saturated fat, 0 trans fat,
20g carbohydrates, 0 cholesterol, 1mg sodium, 1g fiber

SPICED APPLES
(MAKES 4–6 SERVINGS)

⅛ cup low-calorie baking sweetener
⅛ teaspoon ground cinnamon
6 small red apples (about 2 ½ inches diameter)
1½ teaspoons light amber maple syrup
1½ cups dry white wine
¾ cup (6 ounces) apple cider
Dash nutmeg
½ teaspoon finely minced fresh orange peel

Combine sweetener and cinnamon. Roll apples in syrup, then in cinnamon/sweetener mixture. Place apples in a baking dish, and bake at 400 degrees for 15 minutes. Combine wine, cider, nutmeg, and orange peel; heat on low heat. Pour over baked apples and serve.

Approx. 114 calories per serving
<0.5g protein, <0.5g total fat, 0 saturated fat, 0 trans fat,
20g carbohydrates, 0 cholesterol, 5mg sodium, 3g fiber

STRAWBERRIES AMARETTO
(MAKES 8 SERVINGS)

3 pints fresh strawberries
2 cups plain low-fat yogurt
1 teaspoon vanilla extract
¼ cup Amaretto liqueur
Fat-free whipped cream (if desired)

Set aside 8 strawberries for garnish. Hull remaining strawberries and cut into halves. Place strawberry halves in dessert cups. In a bowl combine yogurt, vanilla extract, and liqueur; blend well. Pour over strawberries and garnish each cup with a reserved berry. Add whipped cream if desired.

Approx. 96 calories per serving
4g protein, 0.6g total fat, <0.5 saturated fat, 0 trans fat,
9g carbohydrates, <0.5mg cholesterol, 42mg sodium, 3g fiber

LEMON SHERBET
(MAKES 4–6 SERVINGS)

3 large lemons
½ cup honey
2½ cups water
¼ cup liquid egg whites

Remove zest from lemons, and set aside. Squeeze all 3 lemons to get ⅔ cup of fresh lemon juice, and set juice aside. In a saucepan add zest, honey, and water. Bring to a rapid boil for 5 minutes, then allow to cool to room temperature. Strain lemon juice through a sieve. When honey mixture has cooled, add strained lemon juice, pour into freezer container, and freeze until mushy. When mushy, stir ice crystals from edges of container. Do this every hour for 4 hours, then remove from freezer and whisk until smooth. Beat egg whites to stiffen and fold into whisked lemon mixture. Cover and return to freezer for another 2–3 hours, until mixture has the consistency of packed snow. Serve immediately.

This recipe can also be used to make orange sherbet, substituting oranges for lemons.

Approx. 91 calories per serving
1g protein, 0 total fat, 0 saturated fat, 0 trans fat,
22g carbohydrates, 0 cholesterol, 16mg sodium, 0 fiber

SOUR CREAM AND WALNUT COOKIES
(MAKES 20–25 COOKIES)

Canola oil cooking spray
½ cup trans fat–free canola/olive oil spread
⅔ cup low-calorie baking sweetener
⅔ cup low-fat sour cream
1½ cups all-purpose unbleached flour
1 teaspoon baking soda
½ cup chopped walnuts

Lightly coat two cookie sheets with cooking oil spray. In a bowl combine shortening and sweetener. Use an electric beater on very low to whip mixture into a soft consistency. Add sour cream and whip again for a few seconds to blend. Sift flour and baking soda into sour cream mixture. With a wooden spatula, fold flour and baking soda into mixture until well blended. Add walnuts to dough mixture. Drop 1 tablespoon of dough on the cookie sheet for each cookie. Allow room between cookies. Press cookies flat with a wooden spatula and bake at 350 degrees, until golden brown (about 10–15 minutes). Remove from the oven and allow cookies to cool before serving.

Approx. 82 calories per cookie
3g protein, 3g total fat, 1g saturated fat, 0 trans fat,
5g carbohydrates, 2mg cholesterol, 38mg sodium, <1g fiber

MERINGUE KEY LIME DESSERT CUPS
(MAKES 6–8 SERVINGS)

1½ cups low-calorie baking sweetener
¼ cup cornstarch
¼ teaspoon sodium-free salt substitute
¼ cup + 2 tablespoons fresh Key lime juice
½ cup cold water
¾ cup whole egg substitute
2 tablespoons of a trans fat–free canola/olive oil spread
½ cup of boiling water
2 teaspoons grated fresh lime zest

For Meringue:

½ cup low-calorie baking sweetener
¾ cup egg whites
¼ teaspoon cream of tartar
8 thin slices fresh lime for garnish

Combine sweetener, cornstarch, and salt in a large saucepan. Add lime juice, water, and egg substitute; blend well. Add canola/olive oil spread and slowly blend in boiling water. Heat mixture to boiling over medium heat and cook for 2–3 minutes, stirring constantly. Add in lime zest, remove mixture from heat, and set aside to cool.

Meringue:

Place egg whites in a bowl and whip on low speed until they start to bubble. Turn speed to medium-high; add cream of tartar and whip until mixture holds a peak. Continue whipping on high while gradually adding sweetener. Meringue will stiffen and peak. Fill dessert cups with Key lime mixture and top with a healthy dollop of meringue. Place in a 350-degree oven until meringue lightly browns. Serve warm or cold.

Approx. 58 calories per serving
5g protein, 2g total fat, 0.4g saturated fat, 0 trans fat,
16g carbohydrates, 0 cholesterol, 109mg sodium, 0 fiber

HOMESTYLE APPLE PIE
(MAKES 8 SERVINGS)

For Crust:

1 cup pastry flour
6 tablespoons canola oil
3 tablespoons water
All-purpose flour

For Filling:

6 sweet apples, cored, peeled, and sliced (Red or Yellow Delicious, Gala, or Macintosh)
⅔ cup low-calorie baking sweetener
⅛ teaspoon salt
¾ teaspoon cinnamon
¾ teaspoon nutmeg
1½ tablespoons trans fat–free canola oil/olive oil spread

Crust:

Prepare dough by combining pastry flour with oil and water. Mix well and form into a ball. Use a small amount of all-purpose flour to coat work surface, place dough on surface, and sprinkle a small amount of all-purpose flour on dough to keep it from sticking to the rolling pin. Roll out dough into a flat circle large enough to cover the inside and sides of a 9-inch pie pan.

Filling:

Place sliced apples in a bowl, add sweetener, salt, cinnamon, and nutmeg, and stir to coat apple slices with dried ingredients. Transfer apple mixture to dough-lined pie pan. Spread apples out evenly. Place dots of canola/olive oil spread onto the top of apples and put pie into oven. Bake at 450 degrees for 15 minutes. Reduce oven temperature to 350 degrees, and bake for another 45 minutes. Remove from oven and cool slightly before cutting. Serve warm with fat-free whipped cream if desired.

Approx. 111 calories per serving
1g protein, 2g total fat, 0 saturated fat, 0 trans fat,
23g carbohydrates, 0 cholesterol, 88mg sodium, 3g fiber

TOASTED CRÊPE CUPS WITH FRESH BERRIES IN A LEMON YOGURT SAUCE

(MAKES 4 SERVINGS)

4 (prepared) flat crêpes (use only trans fat–free brands)
Canola oil cooking spray
½ cup + 4 tablespoons low-fat plain yogurt
½ cup fat-free cream cheese
4 teaspoons fresh lemon juice
2 teaspoons non-caloric sweetener
10 pecan halves, chopped
1 cup blueberries, fresh or frozen (thawed)
8 strawberries, hulled and sliced
4 whole strawberries for garnish (optional)
4 fresh mint leaves for garnish (optional)

Invert 4 oven-safe dessert cups on a baking sheet and lightly spray the outside of each cup with cooking oil spray. Form 1 flat crêpe around each dessert cup, folding crêpes down the center to fit cup size better if necessary (crêpes will not adhere completely to cups but will take on enough of its form to give them a cup shape when baked). Spray tops of crêpes very lightly with cooking oil spray and place baking sheet in oven. Bake crêpes until golden brown and crispy (about 6–7 minutes). Remove from oven and allow to cool before removing crêpes from cups. Meanwhile, combine yogurt and cream cheese in a bowl. Stir until well blended. Add in lemon juice and sweetener. Stir until all ingredients are well blended. Add pecans to mixture and gently fold in blueberries and strawberries. Divide mixture into 4 portions and spoon into formed crêpe cups. Garnish with a fresh whole strawberry and a fresh mint leaf if desired.

Approx. 133 calories per serving
5g protein, 3g total fat, 0 saturated fat, 0 trans fat,
16g carbohydrates, 23mg cholesterol, 180mg sodium, 2g fiber

TOASTED SAUTÉED BANANA AND STRAWBERRY CRÊPES
(MAKES 4 SERVINGS)

4 (prepared) flat crêpes (use only trans fat–free brands)
Canola oil cooking spray
2 small bananas, sliced lengthwise
Cinnamon and non-caloric sweetener for sprinkling
4 teaspoons fat-free cream cheese
½ cup fresh strawberries, sliced
⅛ cup raw sliced almonds
Fat-free sour cream for garnish (optional)

Lightly spray a heavy-bottomed skillet with cooking oil and sauté the bananas (sprinkled with cinnamon and sweetener) until lightly browned. Remove from heat and set aside. Spread 1 teaspoon of cream cheese down the center of each crêpe. Place a sautéed banana half on top of the cheese and add strawberries. Fold crêpes over to form a pocket while folding in the ends. Place folded crêpes on a baking sheet lightly sprayed with canola oil cooking spray; also spray tops of crêpes. Sprinkle tops of crêpes with almond slices and sweetener. Place in oven and bake until crêpes are golden brown and crispy (about 7–9 minutes). Serve warm with a dollop of sour cream if desired.

Approx. 119 calories per serving
4g protein, 1g total fat, 0 saturated fat, 0 trans fat,
21g carbohydrates, 5mg cholesterol, 67mg sodium, 4g fiber

FRUITED NUTTY PASTRY ROLLS
(MAKES 20 PIECES)

Canola oil cooking spray
4 tablespoons trans fat–free canola/olive oil spread
¼ cup low-calorie baking sweetener
1 egg
1 teaspoon almond extract
⅔ cup all-purpose unbleached flour, sifted
4 tablespoons natural chunky peanut butter
4 tablespoons low-sugar fruit jam
⅛ cup finely chopped walnuts

Lightly coat a baking sheet with cooking spray. In a bowl beat together canola/olive oil spread and sweetener until soft and fluffy. Crack the egg and separate the yolk from the white; reserve white. Beat the egg yolk and vanilla extract into the spread and sweetener mixture. Add in sifted flour. Stir to mix all ingredients and form firm dough ball. Add in a small amount of extra flour if dough is too soft. Divide the dough in half and roll out each half into a log about 10 inches long. Place both logs on the baking sheet. Lightly spray the handle of a dinner knife with cooking spray. Starting about ⅛ inch from the beginning of each log, use the knife handle to make a channel down the center, stopping about ⅛ inch before the end of the log. Whisk the egg white gently and brush it over each log. Fill the channel with peanut butter and top with jam. Sprinkle with walnut pieces. Chill logs for about 30–45 minutes. Heat oven to 350 degrees and bake chilled logs until they are a light golden brown (about 10–12 minutes). Remove from oven and allow logs to cool until jam sets. Slice each roll diagonally into 10 slices before serving.

Approx. 78 calories per piece
4g protein, 6g total fat, 1g saturated fat, 0 trans fat,
5g carbohydrates, 11mg cholesterol, 50mg sodium, <0.5g fiber

MERINGUE COOKIES
(MAKES 20–24 COOKIES)

1 cup liquid egg whites
Pinch of cream of tartar
¼ cup low-calorie baking sweetener
1 teaspoon white wine vinegar
1 teaspoon vanilla extract

Line 2 cookie trays with parchment paper. Place egg whites in a mixing bowl and slowly whisk on low speed with an electric beater until they begin to bubble. Add cream of tartar and increase speed slightly; whisk until the mixture begins to peak. Increase speed to medium and slowly add sweetener, vinegar, and vanilla extract. Continue whisking until mixture is satiny and firmly holds peak. Ladle a soup spoon-sized portion of mixture onto parchment-lined trays to make 20–24 cookies. Put trays of meringues in an oven preheated to 275 degrees to bake for about 1 hour. Turn off oven and allow cookies to stand in closed oven for an additional hour to dry. When meringues are pierced with a toothpick that comes back dry, they are ready. Transfer cookies to cooling racks to continue to cool.

Approx. 5 calories per cookie
1g protein, 0 total fat, 0 saturated fat, 0 trans fat,
<0.1g carbohydrates, 0 cholesterol, 15mg sodium, 0 fiber

RASPBERRY MERINGUES
(MAKES 30–40 COOKIES)

¾ cup liquid egg whites
½ cup sliced raw almonds
2 tablespoons low-calorie baking sweetener
¼ teaspoon almond extract
⅛ teaspoon sodium-free salt substitute
⅓ cup non-caloric sweetener
⅓ cup low-calorie raspberry jam

Egg whites need to be at room temperature for 30 minutes before use. Line cookie sheets with parchment paper. Combine sliced almonds and 2 tablespoons of sweetener in a food processor or blender, and process until finely ground. In a large bowl add egg whites, almond extract, and salt substitute, and whip on medium speed until mixture begins to bubble. Gradually add ⅓ cup of sweetener a little at a time, increasing speed to high, and whip until mixture forms stiff peaks. Gently fold in almond mixture. Ladle soup spoon-sized portions of mixture onto parchment paper, making about 30–40 cookies. Bake for 20–25 minutes in an oven preheated to 275 degrees. Turn oven off and allow cookies to stand in closed oven for an additional hour to dry. Transfer cookies to cooling racks to continue to cool. When completely cooled, spoon a small amount of raspberry jam into center of each cookie.

Approx. 11 calories per cookie
6g protein, 0.7g total fat, 0 saturated fat, 0 trans fat,
8g carbohydrates, 0 cholesterol, 6mg sodium, .03g fiber

BROWNIES
(MAKES 24 BROWNIES)

*1 ¼ cups cake flour (or substitute a combination of all-purpose flour and
    cornstarch as follows: 2 ½ tablespoons of cornstarch plus enough flour to
    fill 1 ¼ cups)*
½ teaspoon sodium-free salt substitute
¾ teaspoon baking powder
3 tablespoons unsweetened dark baking cocoa
2 ¼ cups low-calorie baking sweetener
1 cup liquid egg substitute
4 tablespoons canola oil
1 tablespoon vanilla extract

Combine all dry ingredients in a large bowl and whisk to incorporate. In a separate bowl combine egg, oil, and vanilla extract. Pour egg
mixture into dry ingredients and mix until batter is smooth and blended. Pour batter into a non-stick 9x13-inch baking pan and spread batter
out evenly over bottom. Place pan on middle shelf in a 300-degree oven.
Bake brownies for roughly 8–10 minutes; the center should spring back
when touched with a finger, or you can insert a tooth pick into the center.
Brownies are done when the toothpick comes out with just a few moist
crumbs on it. Do not overbake brownies or they will be dry. Immediately
remove pan from oven, and allow brownies to cool on cooling rack before cutting

    Approx. 54 calories per brownie
    2g protein, 3g total fat, <0.4g saturated fat, 0 trans fat,
    5g carbohydrates, 0 cholesterol, 33mg sodium, <0.5g fiber

ORANGE MACAROONS
(MAKES 15 COOKIES)

Canola oil cooking spray
½ cup liquid egg whites
2 tablespoons low-calorie baking sweetener
1 teaspoon finely grated fresh orange zest
¼ teaspoon vanilla or orange extract
Dash of salt (optional)
1½ cups sweetened dried flaked coconut

Line a cookie sheet with parchment paper and spray lightly with cooking spray. In a bowl add egg whites, sweetener, zest, extract, salt, and coconut. Stir to incorporate ingredients. Drop tablespoons of mixture onto parchment paper to make about 15 cookies. Allow about 1½ inches between each cookie. Bake in an oven preheated to 325 degrees on the middle oven rack for roughly 15–20 minutes, or until the tops are a pale golden brown. Remove from oven and allow to cool.

Approx. 37 calories per cookie
1g protein, 3g total fat, 2g saturated fat, 0 trans fat,
2g carbohydrates, 0 cholesterol, 11mg sodium, <0.2g fiber

FRESH PINEAPPLE IN SPICY RUM SYRUP
(MAKES 6 SERVINGS)

1 fresh pineapple (roughly 3 pounds)
2½ cups water
½ cup low-calorie baking sweetener
8 slices of fresh ginger
3 tablespoons of dark rum
12 fresh mint leaves
Fat-free whipped cream

Trim top off pineapple and peel. Cut in half, core, and cut each half into ¼-inch slices. Set slices aside. In a large heavy-bottomed skillet, bring water, sweetener, and ginger to a boil. Stir mixture constantly until sweetener dissolves, and continue boiling uncovered for an additional 3–4 minutes. Remove from heat and let stand uncovered for another 10–12 minutes to allow the liquid to be infused with the ginger's flavor. With a slotted spoon remove ginger and discard. Add pineapple slices, cover, and simmer, stirring often, until pineapple looks translucent (about 6–8 minutes). With a slotted spoon remove pineapple to a heat-proof bowl. Boil liquid to a reduction of 1 cup of syrup, stirring constantly (about 8–10 minutes). Add rum to syrup and return to a gentle boil for another 1 minute. Pour syrup over pineapple, allow all to come to room temperature, and then chill for 1 hour. Serve garnished with fresh mint leaves and a dollop of fat-free whipped cream.

Approx. 75 calories per serving
0.5g protein, 0.5g total fat, .05g saturated fat, 0 trans fat,
15g carbohydrates, 0 cholesterol, 1mg sodium, 1g fiber

CHOCOLATE SWEET TREATS
(MAKES ABOUT 40 PIECES)

¾ cup ground flaxseed
3 tablespoons chocolate-flavored whey protein
1½ teaspoons ground cinnamon
½ cup fat-free, sugar-free chocolate syrup
2 tablespoons chunky peanut butter
1 tablespoon unsweetened dark cocoa powder

Mix flaxseed, whey protein, cinnamon, syrup, and peanut butter together in a bowl; stir to blend well. Spoon 35–40 teaspoon-sized portions onto a cookie sheet covered with parchment paper. Lightly sprinkle each treat with a small amount of cocoa powder and refrigerate to chill; let harden for about 2 hours.

Approx. 20 calories per piece
1g protein, 1g total fat, 0.1g saturated fat, 0 trans fat,
1g carbohydrates, <0.1mg cholesterol, 8mg sodium, 1g fiber

HEALTHY CHOCOLATE CUPCAKES
(MAKES 12 CUPCAKES)

1 ¼ cups pastry flour
3 tablespoons ground flaxseed
1 cup low-calorie baking sweetener
½ cup unsweetened dark cocoa
½ teaspoon baking soda
½ teaspoon baking powder
½ teaspoon sodium-free salt substitute
½ cup concentrated pomegranate juice, or other clear concentrated juice
¾ cup vanilla soy milk
3 tablespoons canola oil
⅓ cup chopped walnuts

Mix together flour, flaxseed, sweetener, cocoa, baking soda, baking powder, and salt substitute. Blend all ingredients well with a whisk. Make a well in the center of the mixture. In a separate bowl add juice, soy milk, oil, and ⅔ of the walnuts (reserve ⅓ for garnish). Stir ingredients well and pour mixture into the well of the flour mixture. With a spatula, blend all ingredients until well mixed. Line a 12-cup cupcake pan with paper cupcake liners and fill each liner until almost full. Sprinkle a small amount of the reserved chopped walnuts on top of each cupcake. Place pans in a 350-degree oven on center rack and bake for 18–20 minutes, or until a tooth pick inserted in the center of a cupcake comes out clean. Do not overbake. Allow to cool for 10–15 minutes before serving.

Approx. 135 calories per cupcake
7g protein, 7g total fat, 1g saturated fat, 0 trans fat,
17g carbohydrates, 0 cholesterol, 79mg sodium, 1g fiber

HEALTHY BANANA NUT MUFFINS
(MAKES 12 MUFFINS)

1 cup (8 ounces) of soy flour

2 teaspoons baking powder

2 tablespoons low-calorie baking sweetener

¼ cup finely chopped walnuts

2 medium-sized ripe bananas, mashed

1 teaspoon vanilla extract

1¼ cups vanilla soy milk

¼ cup egg substitute

2 tablespoons canola oil

2 tablespoons dry oatmeal

Line a 12-cup muffin pan with paper muffin cups. Sift soy flour and baking powder together into a mixing bowl. Add sweetener and nuts, and stir to mix ingredients. Make a well in the center of the mix and add bananas, extract, soy milk, egg substitute, and oil. Pour batter into muffin cups, sprinkle tops with oatmeal, and bake in a 350-degree oven for 20–25 minutes, or until muffins are firm and a toothpick inserted into the center of a muffin comes back dry. Remove from oven and allow to cool.

Approx. 100 calories per muffin
5g protein, 6g total fat, 0.6g saturated fat, 0 trans fat,
9g carbohydrates, 0 cholesterol, 22mg sodium, 2g fiber

CARAMELIZED PEARS
(MAKES 6 SERVINGS)

3 ripe Bartlett pears, peeled, cut in half, and cored
3 tablespoons fresh lemon juice
1 tablespoon vanilla extract
3 tablespoons trans fat–free canola/olive oil spread
½ cup low-calorie baking sweetener
8 tablespoons low-fat plain yogurt
6 lemon slices for garnish (optional)

Place pears in a large bowl; add lemon juice and vanilla extract. Gently toss ingredients to coat pears. Melt spread in an oven-safe skillet over medium-high heat. Add sweetener and stir to distribute sweetener evenly in pan. Place pears cut side down in skillet and drizzle remaining lemon juice mixture from bowl over pears. Cook until sweetener begins to dissolve and mixture bubbles, shaking pan often to move mixture around and under pears while cooking. Cook for about 5 minutes. Transfer skillet to oven and bake until pears are soft and juices are golden colored (about 15–20 minutes). Serve pears warm, drizzled with mixture from pan; add a tablespoon of yogurt on the side and garnish with a lemon slice.

Approx. 102 calories per serving
2g protein, 5g total fat, 1.5g saturated fat, 0 trans fat,
14g carbohydrates, 1mg cholesterol, 61mg sodium, 2g fiber

PLUM SORBET
(MAKES 10–12 SERVINGS)

1 pound (about 14) red plums, halved and pitted
6 ounces sweet red sherry
¾ cup water
1½ cups non-caloric sweetener
1 cinnamon stick
1 teaspoon vanilla extract
Zest from half a lemon

Place the freezer canister of an ice cream maker in the freezer. Combine plums, sherry, water, sweetener, cinnamon stick, vanilla extract, and zest in a heavy saucepan and cook, covered, over medium heat, stirring occasionally, until plums fall apart (about 20–30 minutes). Remove cinnamon stick. Place plum mixture in a blender or food processor and process until smooth. Strain pureed mixture through a mesh strainer to separate any remaining large pieces. Allow to cool, then transfer mixture to cold ice cream canister and return to freezer uncovered for about 2 hours. When sorbet is cold, transfer to an airtight freezer container for at least 1 more hour before serving.

Approx. 56 calories per serving
0.6g protein, 0.23 total fat, 0 saturated fat, 0 trans fat,
11g carbohydrates, 0 cholesterol, 1mg sodium, 1g fiber

DARK DOUBLE CHOCOLATE PUDDING
(MAKES 6–8 SERVINGS)

¼ cup egg substitute
3 cups skim milk
⅔ cup low-calorie baking sweetener
¼ cup corn starch
3 tablespoons unsweetened dark cocoa powder
⅛ teaspoon low-sodium salt
½ teaspoon pure vanilla extract
2 ounces dark chocolate chips
Fat-free whipped cream for garnish

Beat egg substitute lightly and set aside. Gradually heat milk over low heat until it begins to bubble. Remove from heat and add sweetener, corn starch, cocoa, and salt. Bring mixture to a boil over medium heat while whisking constantly. When mixture thickens slightly, remove from heat. Slowly add egg substitute to 1 cup of milk mixture (do this so that egg subsitute does not immediately cook) and whisk. Pour egg mixture into remaining milk mixture and return to a boil, whisking constantly. When mixture thickens to pudding consistency, remove from heat and add vanilla extract and chocolate chips. Stir to incorporate, then pour into bowl and cover with plastic wrap. Push wrap down into bowl so it touches top of pudding; this keeps pudding from developing a skin on the top. Refrigerate until ready to serve, and garnish with whipped cream if desired.

Approx. 92 calories per serving
4g protein, 1.7g total fat, 0.39g saturated fat, 0 trans fat,
13g carbohydrates, 2mg cholesterol, 97mg sodium, 0.4g fiber

ORANGE ANGEL FOOD CUPCAKES
(MAKES 6–8 LARGE CUPCAKES)

1½ cups egg whites
1 teaspoon cream of tartar
¼ teaspoon low-sodium salt
1 teaspoon orange extract
Zest and juice from a small orange
¾ cup low-calorie baking sweetener
½ cup + 1 tablespoon cake flour
Fat-free whipped cream and maraschino cherries for garnish

In a mixing bowl beat egg whites with electric beater on high until foamy. Add cream of tartar, salt, orange extract, and orange zest and juice. Beat again until mixture is stiff and peaks. Add sweetener, one cup at a time, while continuing to beat. With a wooden spoon, fold in flour and gently stir to mix. Line a cupcake tin with 6 paper liners and spoon mixture into liners. Bake on the bottom rack of a 350-degree oven for 15–20 minutes or until the center of cupcakes springs back when touched. Remove from oven and allow to cool before serving. Garnish with whipped cream and a maraschino cherry if desired.

Approx. 58 calories per cupcake
6g protein, 0 total fat, 0 saturated fat, 0 trans fat,
8g carbohydrates, 0 cholesterol, 140mg sodium, 0 fiber

Smoothies

NOTE: The delicious smoothies listed below can also be prepared without whey protein.

BLUEBERRY BURST WHEY SMOOTHIE
(MAKES 1 16-OUNCE SERVING)

½ cup cold water
¼ cup fresh or unsweetened frozen blueberries
2 packets non-caloric sweetener
¼ cup plain non-fat yogurt
1 scoop natural-flavored whey protein powder
8 ice cubes
Fat-free whipped cream
Sprinkle of crushed almonds for garnish

In an ice-crushing blender, add water, berries, and sweetener and blend until smooth. Add yogurt and whey, and blend until smooth again. Add ice cubes and chop until crushed. Pour into glass and top with whipped cream and almonds.

Approx. 124 calories per serving
22g protein, 1g total fat, 0 saturated fat, 0 trans fat,
10g carbohydrates, 2mg cholesterol, 88mg sodium, 1g fiber

STRAWBERRY SUNDAE WHEY SMOOTHIE
(MAKES 1 16-OUNCE SERVING)

½ cup cold water
½ cup fresh or unsweetened frozen strawberries
¼ teaspoon vanilla extract
2 packets non-caloric sweetener
¼ cup plain non-fat yogurt
1 scoop natural-flavored whey protein powder
8 ice cubes
Fat-free whipped cream
Fat-free, sugar-free chocolate syrup to drizzle

In an ice-crushing blender, add water, berries, extract, and sweetener, and blend until smooth. Add yogurt and whey, and blend until smooth again. Add ice and chop until crushed. Pour into glass and top with whipped cream and chocolate syrup.

Approx. 134 calories per serving
21g protein, 1g total fat, 0 saturated fat, 0 trans fat,
11g carbohydrates, 2mg cholesterol, 94mg sodium, 2g fiber

CHOCOLATE MOUSSE WHEY SMOOTHIE

(MAKES 1 16-OUNCE SERVING)

½ cup cold water
½ cup plain fat-free yogurt
1 scoop natural-flavored whey protein powder
2 packets non-caloric sweetener
1 tablespoon fat-free, sugar-free chocolate syrup
1 teaspoon almond extract
8 ice cubes
Fat-free whipped cream
Fat-free, sugar-free chocolate syrup to drizzle
Sprinkle of crushed almonds for garnish (optional)

In an ice-crushing blender, add water, yogurt, whey, sweetener, syrup, and almond extract, and blend until smooth. Add ice and chop until crushed. Pour into a glass and top with whipped cream, syrup, and almonds.

Approx. 145 calories per serving
24g protein, 1g total fat, 0 saturated fat, 0 trans fat,
11g carbohydrates, 3mg cholesterol, 148mg sodium, 0 fiber

PINEAPPLE DELIGHT WHEY SMOOTHIE
(MAKES 1 16-OUNCE SERVING)

½ cup cold water
½ cup fresh pineapple, diced
1 teaspoon pineapple extract
2 packets non-caloric sweetener
¼ cup plain non-fat yogurt
1 scoop natural-flavored whey protein powder
8 ice cubes
Fat-free whipped cream
Crushed walnuts for garnish

In an ice-crushing blender, add water, pineapple, pineapple extract, and sweetener, and blend until smooth. Add yogurt and whey, and blend until smooth again. Add ice and chop until crushed. Pour into a glass and top with whipped cream and walnuts.

Approx. 149 calories per serving
20g protein, 1g total fat, 0 saturated fat, 0 trans fat,
16g carbohydrates, 1mg cholesterol, 88mg sodium, 1g fiber

BANANA PEACH VANILLA SOY MILK SMOOTHIE
(MAKES 1 SMOOTHIE)

1 cup light vanilla soy milk
1 medium banana
1 medium peach, pitted and sliced
1 cup ice
1 teaspoon vanilla extract
Non-caloric sweetener

In a blender combine soy milk, banana, peach, and ice. Process to desired consistency; with machine running, add extract and sweetener. Serve immediately.

Approx. 204 calories per smoothie
5g protein, 3g total fat, 0 saturated fat, 0 trans fat,
19g carbohydrates, 0 cholesterol, 2mg sodium, 3g fiber

CHOCOLATE RASPBERRY SOY MILK SMOOTHIE
(MAKES 1 SMOOTHIE)

1 cup light chocolate soy milk
1 medium banana
1 cup frozen unsweetened raspberries
1 cup ice
1 teaspoon vanilla extract
Non-caloric sweetener to taste

In a blender combine soy milk, banana, raspberries, and ice. Process to desired consistency; with machine running, add extract and sweetener. Serve immediately.

Approx. 317 calories per smoothie
8g protein, 4g total fat, 0.5g saturated fat, 0 trans fat,
66g carbohydrates, 0 cholesterol, 136mg sodium, 9g fiber

MELON MADNESS WHEY SMOOTHIE
(MAKES 1 16-OUNCE SERVING)

½ cup cold water
½ (5–6-inch) fresh cantaloupe
2 packets non-caloric sweetener
¼ cup plain non-fat yogurt
1 scoop natural-flavored whey protein powder
8 ice cubes
Fat-free whipped cream
Crushed almonds for garnish

In an ice-crushing blender, add water, cantaloupe, sweetener, yogurt, and whey, and blend until smooth. Add ice and chop until crushed. Pour into glass and top with whipped cream and almonds.

Approx. 204 calories per serving
22g protein, 1g total fat, 0 saturated fat, 0 trans fat,
27g carbohydrates, 1mg cholesterol, 111mg sodium, 2g fiber

Appetizers, Dips, and Snack Foods

Appetizers

ROASTED GARLIC
(MAKES 4–5 SERVINGS)

1 elephant jumbo garlic head
Extra-virgin olive oil to drizzle
Dry seasonings of choice (optional)

Holding entire head of garlic, cut off the top leaf points of each clove to expose a small portion of the clove. Keep the remainder of leaves intact around the body of the garlic head. Place trimmed garlic head in a tight-fitting oven-safe bowl, trimmed side up. Drizzle a small amount of olive oil over the top of the head and down around the sides. Sprinkle with your favorite seasoning (optional). Place garlic on middle rack of oven and bake at 400 degrees for 20–30 minutes, or until cloves are soft and a light golden brown. Remove from oven and spread garlic on crusty bread, or add to vegetables, omelets, or pasta.

Approx. 59 calories per serving
3g protein, 0.2g total fat, <1g saturated fat, 0 trans fat,
13g carbohydrates, 0 cholesterol, 7mg sodium, 1g fiber

STUFFED GRAPE LEAVES (DOLMAS)
(MAKES 20 SERVINGS)

3 tablespoons extra-virgin olive oil
1 cup chopped red onion
½ cup chopped scallions
1 cup basmati rice
4 garlic cloves, minced
1 teaspoon ground cumin
½ teaspoon freshly ground pepper
2 cups low-sodium vegetable broth
¼ cup chopped fennel
¼ cup chopped dill
¼ cup finely chopped parsley
2 tablespoons dried mint
1 (16-ounce) jar grape leaves
2 cups water

For Yogurt Sauce:
2 cups plain non-fat yogurt
4 scallions, minced
1 clove garlic, minced
1 teaspoon salt

In a skillet over medium heat add 1 tablespoon oil, onions, and scallions; cook until soft and transparent. Add rice, and cook until grains are slightly browned, stirring constantly. Add garlic, cumin, pepper, and vegetable broth. Reduce heat to simmer, cover, and cook until rice is tender and all liquid is absorbed. Allow rice to cool, then stir in fennel, dill, parsley, and mint. Set aside. Drain grape leaves and cover with water; bring to a rolling boil. Blanch leaves for 1–2 minutes, drain, and allow to cool. With leaf shiny side down, fill with mixture and roll starting at the stem and folding in sides. Repeat until all 20 leaves are filled. Line a heavy-bottomed pan with 10 of the unfilled grape leaves. Pack the rolled leaves in tightly side by side, seam side down. Top rolled leaves with lemon slices and cover lemon slices with remaining unfilled grape leaves. Mix together 2 cups water and remaining olive oil and pour over grape leaf rolls. Place an object like a heavy plate on top of rolls to help hold them below the water level during cooking, and simmer for about 1 hour, checking to make sure they haven't boiled dry. Remove pan from stove and allow to cool. Remove rolls from pan and chill. Serve chilled or at room temperature, garnished with lemon wedges or yogurt sauce.

Yogurt Sauce:

Mix together plain yogurt, scallions, garlic, and salt to taste. Chill until ready to serve.

Approx. 59 calories per serving
1g protein, 2g total fat, 0.2g saturated fat, 0 trans fat,
9g carbohydrates, 0 cholesterol, 123mg sodium, 1g fiber

TOMATO AND GARLIC BRUSCHETTA
(MAKES ENOUGH FOR 8 SERVINGS)

8 slices (½-inch thick) of a French baguette or a crusty whole grain bread
1 teaspoon extra-virgin olive oil
1¼ cups chopped plum tomatoes
1½ teaspoons minced garlic
1 teaspoon balsamic vinegar
½ teaspoon dried basil
¼ teaspoon of non-caloric sweetener
¼ teaspoon ground pepper

Place slices on ungreased baking sheet. Brush each slice with olive oil and bake at 500 degrees for 3–4 minutes until golden brown. Combine tomatoes, garlic, vinegar, basil, sweetener, and pepper in a small bowl. Mix well and spoon mixture over bread slices.

Approx. 57 calories per serving
2.5g protein, 0.7g total fat, 0.4g saturated fat, 0 trans fat,
11g carbohydrates, 0 cholesterol, 106mg sodium, 1g fiber

TOMATO AND FRESH PARMESAN CHEESE BRUSCHETTA
(MAKES 8 SLICES)

8 slices (½-inch thick) of a French baguette or crusty whole grain bread
2 cloves garlic, finely minced
1 teaspoon extra-virgin olive oil
1 small onion, diced
1 medium tomato, diced
Pinch dried oregano, crumbled
Pinch freshly ground pepper
2 tablespoons freshly grated Parmesan cheese

Scantly brush slices of bread on both sides with oil, then toast. Remove from oven and evenly distribute garlic on one side of bread. Rub garlic into bread with handle of knife and set aside; keep warm. Heat teaspoon of oil in skillet, add onions, and lightly sauté until golden brown. Remove from heat. Preheat broiler. Combine onion, tomatoes, oregano, and pepper; spread evenly over garlic bread and sprinkle with cheese. Place bread with cheese under broiler for 1 minute until lightly browned. Serve immediately.

Approx. 70 calories per serving
3g protein, 1.7g total fat, 0.3g saturated fat, 0 trans fat,
13g carbohydrates, 1mg cholesterol, 127mg sodium, 1g fiber

ITALIAN CROSTINI
(MAKES APPROXIMATELY 25–27 SERVINGS)

1 French baguette roughly 10–12 inches long, cut into ½-inch thick slices
Extra-virgin olive oil cooking spray
2½ teaspoons fresh garlic paste
Minced dry or fresh basil, parsley, or chives
Salt and freshly ground pepper to taste

Lightly spray both sides of each slice with a scant amount of olive oil spray. Rub a scant amount of garlic paste onto one side of each slice, then slightly sprinkle herb of choice over garlic. Add salt and pepper to taste. Place slices on a non-stick cookie sheet and place in a 375-degree oven on middle rack to bake until slices are a light golden brown (about 3–5 minutes). Serve as is or add your favorite topping (smoked mozzarella, chopped fresh tomatoes, chopped black olives, roasted garlic, etc.) if desired.

Approx. 41 calories per serving
1g protein, 0.2g total fat, 0.03g saturated fat, 0 trans fat,
10g carbohydrates, 0 cholesterol, 101mg sodium, 1g fiber

MUSHROOM CROSTINI
(MAKES 4 SERVINGS)

1 (10–12 inch) loaf of crusty whole grain bread
Olive oil cooking spray
1½ tablespoons trans fat–free canola/olive oil spread
1 tablespoon extra-virgin olive oil
3 tablespoons minced shallots
2 tablespoons freshly minced garlic
4 cups assorted mushrooms (such as crimini, shiitake, button, and
    portobello), sliced
½ cup sherry
1 tablespoon freshly chopped parsley
1 teaspoon freshly chopped thyme
Salt and freshly ground pepper to taste
Freshly grated Parmesan cheese for garnish (optional)

Slice bread loaf into 8 thick slices. Lightly spray slices on both sides with olive oil spray and place on a non-stick baking sheet. Bake until slices are crispy and golden brown. Allow canola/olive oil spread to come to room temperature. In a large skillet heat olive oil, add shallots and garlic, and cook until soft. Add mushrooms and sherry to garlic mixture, and cook until mushrooms are tender and most of the liquid has evaporated (gently stir during cooking to blend flavors). When mushrooms are soft, blend in canola/olive oil spread, parsley, thyme, and salt and pepper to taste. Spoon mushroom mixture onto the toasted bread slices, and sprinkle with scant amounts of Parmesan cheese if desired.

Approx. 115 calories per serving
2g protein, 7g total fat, 1g saturated fat, 0 trans fat,
15g carbohydrates, 0 cholesterol, 38mg sodium, 2g fiber

ANTIPASTI

(MAKES 10–15 SERVINGS)

Antipasti means "before the pasta" (traditionally, pasta is the first main course in Italian cuisine). Antipasti tend to include a number of different appetizers laid out on one large platter.

Fruits (choose whatever is in season), cut into manageable pieces
Cheese (use soft and hard, and spicy and mild, cheeses, leaving some in whole wedges and slicing or chunking others)
Seafood (try large to jumbo cooked shrimp, tails on but otherwise shelled; cooked calamari; steamed clams; mussels; smoked oysters; smoked fish)
Other items (try adding marinated artichokes, black and green olives of various flavors, oil-soaked and seasoned sundried tomatoes, roasted peppers, pickled pearl onions, and bread sticks with thin slices of prosciutto wrapped around the tips; use any red fatty meats sparingly)

Use a large platter for presentation (about 15x15 inches), and place items in some semblance of order: fruits by cheese, cheese by meats, pickled items near each other, etc. Make sure all items are drained of liquid before adding to platter. Serve your antipasti with a tray of crunchy whole grain bread or bread sticks.

Dips

CHILLED AVOCADO DIP
(MAKES I CUP)

2 tablespoons lemon juice
2 tablespoons tahini paste
1 large ripe avocado, halved, pitted, and peeled
¼ cup freshly chopped parsley
1 tablespoon extra-virgin olive oil
⅛ cup chopped onion
3 cloves garlic, peeled and chopped
3 tablespoons low-calorie mayonnaise
⅛ teaspoon cayenne pepper
Salt and freshly ground pepper to taste
Dash of paprika

Blend lemon juice and tahini paste, then add avocados, parsley, olive oil, onion, garlic, mayonnaise, cayenne, and salt and pepper to taste. Blend until smooth, transfer to serving bowl, and chill. When ready to serve, sprinkle with paprika.

Approx. 90 calories per 2 tablespoons
1g protein, 9g total fat, 1.3g saturated fat, 0 trans fat,
3g carbohydrates, 2g cholesterol, 52mg sodium, 1g fiber

HUMMUS DIP
(MAKES 1½ CUPS)

1 (19-ounce) can chickpeas, drained, ¼ cup liquid reserved
¼ cup tahini paste
2 cloves garlic, peeled and chopped
6 tablespoons lemon juice
Salt and freshly ground pepper to taste
Drizzle of extra-virgin olive oil
1 tablespoon finely chopped fresh mint

In food processor, process chickpeas, half of liquid, tahini paste, garlic, lemon juice, and salt and pepper until smooth; should be the consistency of butter. Place on serving plate, drizzle with olive oil, and garnish with mint.

Approx. 79 calories per 2 tablespoons
2g protein, 6g total fat, 0.3g saturated fat, 0 trans fat,
5g carbohydrates, 0 cholesterol, 46mg sodium, 1g fiber

GREEK FETA AND WALNUT DIP
(MAKES 2 CUPS)

½ pound feta cheese
2 tablespoons extra-virgin olive oil
⅔ cup low-fat milk
1 cup finely ground walnuts
Pinch of cayenne pepper
2 tablespoons minced parsley

Drain feta cheese, then combine all ingredients in a food processor and process until smooth. Let mixture stand for 1 hour before serving.

Approx. 88 calories per tablespoon
4g protein, 7.7g total fat, 2.5g saturated fat, 0 trans fat,
2g carbohydrates, 13mg cholesterol, 164mg sodium, <0.5g fiber

GREEK BEAN DIP
(MAKES 3¾ CUPS)

2 (15-ounce) cans Great Northern beans, rinsed and drained
4-ounce package of light cream cheese
4 ounces feta cheese
3 cloves minced garlic
2 tablespoons lemon juice
1 tablespoon chopped fresh oregano
½ teaspoon ground pepper
¼ teaspoon salt
½ cup deseeded and finely chopped tomato
¼ cup sliced ripe olives

In a food processor or blender, process beans, cream cheese, feta cheese, garlic, lemon juice, oregano, pepper, and salt until smooth. Transfer mixture to a 1½-quart baking dish, cover, and bake at 350 degrees for 25 minutes, or until heated through. Remove from heat, sprinkle tomato and olives over dip, and serve.

Approx. 23 calories per 1 tablespoon
2g protein, 0.7g total fat, <0.5g saturated fat, 0 trans fat,
2g carbohydrates, 1mg cholesterol, 51mg sodium, <0.5g fiber

HERB CUCUMBER YOGURT DIP
(MAKES 2 CUPS)

1 English cucumber
Salt to taste
2 cloves garlic, chopped
2 teaspoons white wine vinegar
2 tablespoons extra-virgin olive oil
2 cups plain low-fat yogurt
2 teaspoons dill
2 teaspoons dried mint
Freshly ground pepper to taste
2 tablespoons chopped fresh mint

Peel and slice cucumbers (if very seedy, remove seeds). Place in bowl and sprinkle with a little salt; let sit for about 15 minutes to draw out water. In a separate bowl, mash garlic into a paste; add pinch of salt, vinegar, and oil, and stir. Add yogurt, dill, and dried mint, and mix well. Rinse salt from cucumber slices and pat dry, removing any excess water. Combine cucumbers with yogurt mixture; add salt and freshly ground pepper to taste. Garnish with fresh chopped mint and serve.

Approx. 16 calories per ⅛ cup
<0.5g protein, 1g total fat, <0.5g saturated fat, 0 trans fat,
1g carbohydrates, 2mg cholesterol, 7mg sodium, 0 fiber

ROASTED PEPPER DIP
(MAKES 1½ CUPS)

4 large red bell peppers
2 cloves garlic, peeled and minced
1 tablespoon red wine vinegar
3 tablespoons extra-virgin olive oil
Salt and freshly ground pepper to taste

Wash peppers and pat dry. Place on moderately hot grill, turning often until skin is charred and blistered (about 15–20 minutes). Remove from grill and let peppers cool. Rub off blackened skins. Cut each pepper in half, remove stalk and seeds, and cut into ½-inch strips. In a food processor add vinegar and peppers, and pulse, adding oil slowly until peppers are smooth. Transfer pepper mixture from processor to a bowl. Mash garlic and stir into pepper mixture; add salt and pepper to taste.

Approx. 22 calories per 1 tablespoon
<0.2g protein, 2g total fat, <0.2g saturated fat, 0 trans fat,
2g carbohydrates, 0 cholesterol, 0.5mg sodium, 0.5g fiber

HUMMUS WITH TAHINI DIP
(MAKES ABOUT 2 CUPS)

4 cups canned chickpeas, rinsed and drained
3 tablespoons tahini paste
3 tablespoons freshly squeezed lemon juice
4 cloves garlic, crushed into a paste
Salt to taste
1 tablespoon chopped fresh cilantro
4 tablespoons extra-virgin olive oil

Puree chickpeas in a food processor or blender. Blend together the ta-hini, lemon juice, garlic, and salt. Combine this with the chickpeas and blend until it becomes a smooth paste. Serve garnished with cilantro and drizzled with olive oil.

Approx. 84 calories per tablespoon
3g protein, 4.5g total fat, 1g saturated fat, 0 trans fat,
8g carbohydrates, 0 cholesterol, 150mg sodium, 3g fiber

Quick and Easy Snacks

- Any type of fresh fruit or raw vegetable

Nutritional values depend on type of fruit or vegetable choices.

- 10–20 raw almonds or walnuts with 8-ounce glass of water

Approx. 140 calories
5g protein, 12g total fat, 0.8g saturated fat, 0 trans fat,
4g carbohydrates, 0 cholesterol, 0 sodium, 4g fiber

- Whey protein smoothies
  - Blueberry Burst (page 329)
  - Strawberry Sundae (page 330)
  - Chocolate Mousse (page 331)
  - Pineapple Delight (page 332)
  - Melon Madness (page 333)

For nutritional values see page numbers listed above.

- A fresh raw cucumber with skin intact, quartered and sprinkled with herbs such as garlic powder, salt, onion powder, freshly ground pepper, fresh or dried dill, fresh or dried chives, or a combination

Approx. 39 calories
2g protein, 0.4g total fat, <0.1g saturated fat, 0 trans fat,
9g carbohydrates, 0 cholesterol, 6mg sodium, 3g fiber

- A fresh ripe tomato, sliced and seasoned with fresh or dried basil, dried cilantro, garlic powder, salt, freshly ground pepper, dried thyme, marjoram, or a combination

Approx. 38 calories
2g protein, 0.6g total fat, < 0.1g saturated fat, 0 trans fat,
8g carbohydrates, 0 cholesterol, 16mg sodium, 2g fiber

- Popcorn rice cake (trans fat–free) with 1 tablespoon fresh hummus

Approx. 61 calories
2g protein, 1g total fat, 0.2g saturated fat, 0 trans fat,
11g carbohydrates, 0 cholesterol, 82mg sodium, 0.2g fiber

- A raw apple with skin intact, sliced, and 2 teaspoons fresh peanut butter thinly spread onto slices

Approx. 139 calories
2g protein, 6g total fat, 0.8g saturated fat, 0 trans fat,
23g carbohydrates, 0 cholesterol, 37mg sodium, 5g fiber

- 2 Bavarian (no salt added) pretzels (trans fat–free)

Approx. 100 calories
2g protein, 0 total fat, 0 saturated fat, 0 trans fat,
20g carbohydrates, 0 cholesterol, 20mg sodium, 3 fiber

- 1 (3–4 ounce) cup sugar-free, fat-free Jello with 2 tablespoons fat-free whipped cream

Approx. 15 calories
2g protein, 0 total fat, 0 saturated fat, 0 trans fat,
1g carbohydrates, 0 cholesterol, 45mg sodium, 0 fiber

- 1 fat free, no-sugar-added Fudgsicle

Approx. 40 calories
1g protein, 1g total fat, 0.5g saturated fat, 0 trans fat,
9g carbohydrates, 0 cholesterol, 45mg sodium, 2g fiber

Spices, Sauces, Marinades, and Dressings

Spices

MIXED SPICES
(MAKES ABOUT 2 TABLESPOONS)

2 teaspoons ground allspice
1 teaspoon ground cinnamon
1 teaspoon ground cloves
1 teaspoon ground coriander
1 teaspoon ground cumin
¼ teaspoon freshly ground pepper

Combine ingredients and store in a small jar with a tight lid in a cool dry place away from light.

HARISSA (RED PEPPER SPICE)
(MAKES ABOUT ⅔ CUP)

Tunisian kitchens are noted for the spiciness of their food, which comes from a hot pepper sauce called "harissa." The sauce adds piquancy to all types of stews as well as couscous. If you are brave enough, you can even eat it on its own as a spread on bread. Commercial harissa is imported from North Africa and is available in tubes in most gourmet stores where couscous is sold.

½ cup ground fresh cayenne
5 cloves fresh garlic, peeled and crushed
2 tablespoons finely ground caraway seeds
1 tablespoon water
¼ cup cumin
1 teaspoon coriander seed
2 tablespoons salt
½ cup extra-virgin olive oil

Mix all spices together in a mortar. Add crushed garlic and salt to spice mixture and mash together to form a paste. Put paste into a jar and add water and ¼ cup of olive oil; mix well. Spoon remaining olive oil over the top, cover tightly, and refrigerate. It keeps for months.

SPICE RUB
(MAKES ENOUGH FOR 1 POUND OF FISH)

2 tablespoons curry powder
1 tablespoon cumin powder
1 teaspoon sugar
½ teaspoon salt
½ teaspoon paprika
¼ teaspoon cardamom

Combine ingredients and sprinkle fish before cooking.

CHICKEN RUB
(MAKES ENOUGH FOR A 3–4 POUND ROASTER)

1 tablespoon Dijon mustard
1 tablespoon dark spicy mustard
2 cloves garlic, finely minced
1 tablespoon extra-virgin olive oil
1 teaspoon dried thyme
Salt and freshly ground pepper to taste

Combine all ingredients, stir well to incorporate flavors, and rub mixture inside chicken cavity as well as over outside of chicken. Place chicken in refrigerator and marinate for 2–3 hours before roasting.

Sauces

ORANGE GINGER SAUCE
(MAKES 4 SERVINGS)

Juice from 3 fresh oranges
¼ cup light mayonnaise
2 tablespoons prepared fresh horseradish
¼ teaspoon honey
¼ teaspoon ground ginger
1 tablespoon extra-virgin olive oil
Salt and freshly ground pepper to taste
Generous pinch of all-purpose flour

Combine orange juice, mayonnaise, horseradish, honey, ginger, oil, and salt and pepper in a small saucepan. Whisk to blend on low heat. When sauce begins to simmer, whisk in flour. Cook for 1–2 minutes, whisking constantly, until sauce is smooth.

Approx. 60 calories per serving
0 protein, 5g total fat, 0 saturated fat, 0 trans fat,
5g carbohydrates, 0 cholesterol, 155mg sodium, 0 fiber

THICK POMEGRANATE MOLASSES
(MAKES 1 CUP)

3 cups fresh pomegranate juice

In a 1½ quart saucepan bring 3 cups of juice to a boil over medium heat. Reduce heat and simmer, uncovered, stirring occasionally and skimming the froth, until juice is reduced to 1 cup. Cool, bottle, and store in refrigerator.

Approx. 255 calories per 1 cup
3g protein, 0 fat, 0 saturated fat, 0 trans fat,
63g carbohydrates, 0 cholesterol, 0 sodium, 0 fiber

SPICY GARLICKY PESTO SAUCE
(MAKES 4 SERVINGS)

¼ cup extra-virgin olive oil
4 cloves garlic, chopped
¼ teaspoon red hot pepper flakes
Salt and freshly ground pepper to taste

In a medium-sized skillet over medium heat, warm olive oil. Add garlic and sauté until translucent. Add hot pepper flakes and simmer on very low heat for 3–5 minutes. Serve with your favorite pasta. Garnish with grated cheese if desired.

This sauce is also great on pizza.

Approx. 110 calories per serving
0 protein, 14g total fat, 1.5g saturated fat, 0 trans fat,
1g carbohydrates, 0 cholesterol, 1mg sodium, 0 fiber

SUNDRIED TOMATO PESTO
(MAKES 2 CUPS)

1 cup sundried tomatoes
2 cups boiling water
¼ cup + ½ tablespoon extra-virgin olive oil
5 cloves garlic
¼ cup pine nuts
½ cup fresh basil
½ cup Italian parsley

Combine boiling water and sundried tomatoes, and let stand till tomatoes soften (about 10–15 minutes). Drain and reserve 1 cup of liquid. In a medium skillet heat ½ tablespoon oil over medium-high heat. Add garlic and sauté, stirring often for about 1 minute. Remove from heat. In a food processor, process the garlic, tomatoes, reserved liquid, pine nuts, basil, parsley, and remaining ¼ cup olive oil. Serve over pasta.

This sauce is also great on pizza.

Approx. 50 calories per tablespoon
1g protein, 3.5g total fat, 0.6g saturated fat, 0 trans fat,
2g carbohydrates, 0 cholesterol, 23mg sodium, 1g fiber

SPICY PISTACHIO PESTO
(MAKES 4 SERVINGS)

½ small hot cherry pepper, seeded
3 cloves garlic, peeled
2 medium sweet red peppers, roasted
¼ cup dry-roasted pistachios
⅓ cup extra-virgin olive oil
¼ cup fresh grated Parmesan cheese
Salt and freshly ground pepper to taste

In a food processor combine hot pepper, garlic, red peppers, and pistachios. Season with salt and pepper, and pulse while adding olive oil a little at a time until it forms a smooth consistency. Transfer to a bowl and blend in cheese.

This sauce is a great topping for fish.

Approx. 233 calories per serving
4g protein, 23g total fat, 3g saturated fat, 0 trans fat,
5g carbohydrates, 5mg cholesterol, 113mg sodium, 1g fiber

BASIL PESTO SAUCE
(MAKES I CUP OF SAUCE)

⅓ cup pine nuts, toasted
2½ cups fresh basil leaves
1 teaspoon lemon juice
Dash of salt
4 cloves garlic
½ cup extra-virgin olive oil
¼ cup grated Parmesan cheese
¼ cup grated Pecorino Romano cheese
Freshly ground pepper to taste

In a small skillet toast pine nuts over medium heat for 1–2 minutes. Remove from heat and set aside. Cut basil leaves into strips. Combine lemon juice, salt, and garlic in a mortar and mash into a paste. Add pine nuts and continue to mash until nuts are ground. Add basil strips a few at a time, gradually grounding them into nut mixture. Add a splash of olive oil and mix until paste becomes loose. Add grated Parmesan cheese, pepper, and remaining olive oil as needed to form into desirable consistency.

Sauce can be kept refrigerated for a few days if stored in a jar with a tight-fitting lid. If doing this add a small amount of olive oil on top of sauce. However, pesto is best if used immediately.

This sauce goes a long way: one spoonful of pesto is all that is needed to flavor minestrone, vegetables, grilled chicken, fish, or pasta.

Approx. 75 calories per tablespoon
2g protein, 7g total fat, 1.2g saturated fat, 0 trans fat,
2g carbohydrates, 5mg cholesterol, 135mg sodium, <1g fiber

SARDINE PASTA SAUCE

(MAKES 4 SERVINGS)

8–10 small black olives, coarsely chopped
1 (3.75-ounce) tin of sardines in olive oil
2 cloves fresh garlic, pressed
Red hot pepper flakes to taste
¼ cup extra-virgin olive oil
¼ cup finely chopped cilantro
Salt and freshly ground pepper to taste

Combine all the ingredients and mix until sardines are broken into small pieces. Toss with cooked pasta of choice. Add salt and pepper to taste and serve.

Approx. 186 calories per serving
5g protein, 19g total fat, 2.4g saturated fat, 0 trans fat,
<1g carbohydrates, 13mg cholesterol, 121mg sodium, <0.5g fiber

RED CLAM SAUCE
(MAKES 4 SERVINGS)

½ cup white wine
3 cloves garlic, crushed
48 small hard shell clams
1 onion, chopped
2 tablespoons extra-virgin olive oil
2 cups diced plum tomatoes
3 tablespoons chopped fresh basil
1 tablespoon chopped fresh oregano
¼ teaspoon red hot pepper flakes
Salt and freshly ground pepper to taste
1 teaspoon chopped parsley

In a large pot, cook wine, garlic, and clams in small amount of water until shells open. Remove clams from shells. In a skillet add olive oil and onion and sauté. Add tomatoes, season with basil, oregano, and pepper flakes, and cook for 8 minutes. Add clams in their juices and salt and pepper to taste, and cook for another 2–3 minutes. Serve over pasta and garnish with parsley.

Approx. 99 calories per serving
15g protein, 8.5g total fat, <1g saturated fat, 0 trans fat,
8g carbohydrates, 26mg cholesterol, 68mg sodium, 1g fiber

ANCHOVY AND GARLIC SAUCE
(MAKES 4 SERVINGS)

6 tablespoons extra-virgin olive oil
Oil from anchovies
6 cloves fresh garlic, pressed
2-ounce tin of anchovy fillets packed in oil, drained and chopped
Red hot pepper flakes to taste
2 tablespoons cilantro or parsley, finely chopped
6 tablespoons freshly grated Romano cheese
Salt and freshly ground pepper to taste

Combine oil and garlic in a skillet over medium heat and cook about 1–2 minutes. Add anchovies, cook about 30 seconds, and remove from heat. Add in hot pepper flakes and cilantro or parsley. Add to pasta of choice or use as pizza sauce and serve. Add salt and pepper if needed.

This sauce is also great as a pizza sauce.

Approx. 189 calories per serving
3g protein, 18g total fat, 2g saturated fat, 0 trans fat,
1g carbohydrates, 13mg cholesterol, 387mg sodium, 0 fiber

SIMPLY GREAT MARINARA SAUCE
(MAKES 9 CUPS)

½ cup yellow onion, finely chopped
6 cloves garlic, finely minced
3 tablespoons extra-virgin olive oil
2 (28-ounce) cans tomato puree with no salt added
1 (28-ounce) can crushed tomatoes
1 tablespoon tomato paste
½ teaspoon dried basil
2½ cups water
1 cup low-sodium, fat-free chicken broth
1 teaspoon low-calorie baking sweetener
¼ teaspoon crushed red pepper flakes
Salt and freshly ground pepper to taste

Sauté onions and garlic in olive oil over medium heat until soft; do not brown. Add tomato puree, crushed tomatoes, tomato paste, and basil. Stir to blend flavors. Add water, broth, sweetener, red pepper flakes, and salt and pepper, then bring mixture to a boil, cover, reduce heat to low, and simmer for 1 hour. Store unused sauce (in a sealed container) in the freezer for up to 3–4 months.

Approx. 74 calories per ½ cup sauce
17g protein, 3g total fat, <0.4g saturated fat, 0 trans fat,
12.4g carbohydrates, <0.1mg cholesterol, 131mg sodium, 2g fiber

SIMPLE TOMATO PASTA SAUCE
(MAKES 6–8 SERVINGS)

1½ pounds fresh tomatoes or 1 (28-ounce) can peeled tomatoes
6 cloves fresh garlic, finely chopped
6 tablespoons extra-virgin olive oil
10 fresh basil leaves, chopped
Salt and freshly ground pepper to taste
1 large carrot, finely chopped
1 large onion, finely chopped
1 stalk celery, finely chopped
1 teaspoon finely chopped parsley
½ teaspoon hot red pepper flakes

If using fresh tomatoes, place them in a large pot of water and bring to a boil. Remove from heat, rinse tomatoes under cold water, and immediately peel off skins. This method allows you to easily remove the skins from the tomatoes. Cut peeled tomatoes in chunks and set aside. If using canned tomatoes, drain off liquid and reserve (to be used later if sauce is too thick). In a large skillet over medium-high heat, lightly sauté garlic in oil, then add basil, tomatoes, salt and pepper to taste, carrots, onion, celery, parsley, and hot pepper flakes; cook at medium-high heat for 2–3 minutes. Reduce heat to low and simmer for about 20–25 minutes, stirring often to blend ingredients.

Approx. 119 calories per serving
1g protein, 11g total fat, 1g saturated fat, 0 trans fat,
7g carbohydrates, 0 cholesterol, 15mg sodium, 2g fiber

Marinades and Dressings

GINGER GARLIC MARINADE
(MAKES ENOUGH FOR 1½ POUNDS FISH, POULTRY, OR MEAT)

3 tablespoons extra-virgin olive oil
2 tablespoons low-sodium soy sauce
2 tablespoons fresh lime juice
1 tablespoon ground ginger
1 tablespoon finely chopped fresh garlic
½ teaspoon dry mustard

Combine all ingredients and stir to blend. Place fish, poultry, or meat in a container and cover with marinade. Cover with a tight-fitting lid and turn container upside down several times to coat all pieces with marinade. Place in refrigerator for a minimum of 30 minutes, up to several hours. Remove fish or meat from marinade when ready to cook and discard marinade.

GREAT FISH MARINADE
(MAKES ENOUGH FOR 1½ POUNDS OF FISH)

Juice from 2 fresh large limes
1 tablespoon extra-virgin olive oil
2 tablespoons low-sodium soy sauce
2 cloves fresh garlic, finely chopped
½ cup dry vermouth
2 tablespoons fresh mint leaves, minced

Combine all of the ingredients in a small bowl and whisk to blend. Set aside. Score skin of fish and place in a tightly sealable container in a single layer. Pour marinade over fish and turn to coat both sides. Cover and refrigerate for 2–3 hours, turning container upside down several times while marinating to coat fish. Remove fish when ready to cook and discard marinade.

YOGURT DRESSING
(MAKES 1 CUP)

1 cup plain yogurt
Crushed garlic or spearmint to taste

Mix garlic or spearmint into yogurt, to taste.

Approx. 160 calories per 1 cup
9g protein, 8g fat, 4g saturated fat, 0 trans fat,
13g carbohydrates, 0 cholesterol, 160mg sodium, 0 fiber

LEMON DRESSING
(MAKES ABOUT ½ CUP OF DRESSING)

¼ cup extra-virgin olive oil
¼ cup fresh-squeezed lemon juice
1 medium garlic clove, crushed to a paste
Scant pinch of salt
Freshly ground pepper to taste

Combine all ingredients in a bowl and mix well.

Approx. 61 calories per tablespoon
<0.1g protein, 7g total fat, 0.7g saturated fat, 0 trans fat,
1g carbohydrates, 0 cholesterol, 0.1mg sodium, 0 fiber

SICILIAN DRESSING
(MAKES 1 CUP)

¼ cup water
⅔ cup extra-virgin olive oil
Juice from 1 lemon
2 cloves garlic, sliced
½ cup chopped fresh parsley
1 teaspoon oregano

Bring water to a boil, and pour into a bowl. Add olive oil and beat. Add lemon juice, garlic, parsley, and oregano, and beat again until well mixed. Place mixture in a double boiler and cook for additional 5 minutes, stirring constantly. Use as fish topper, or let cool and serve over salad.

Approx. 80 calories per tablespoon
0 protein, 9g total fat, 1.2g saturated fat, 0 trans fat,
0 carbohydrates, 0 cholesterol, 0 sodium, 0 fiber

APPENDICES

APPENDIX A
The Atherogenic Metabolic Stew

If you ask most people what the cause of heart disease is, they'll say cholesterol. However, there are many other risk factors that increase your likelihood of developing heart disease that you can measure with a blood test.

First of all, cholesterol may be good or bad. Good (HDL) cholesterol helps to remove bad (LDL) cholesterol from our arteries. Triglycerides are another lipid, or fat, which can contribute to plaque buildup in our arteries.

Other metabolic risk factors that increase our risk of cardiovascular disease include:

- *Homocysteine*: a protein in the blood that has been linked to cardiovascular disease because of the damage it does to the lining of the blood vessels. It also leads to enhanced clotting. Although homocysteine predicts an increased risk of cardiovascular disease, it has not been demonstrated that lowering homocysteine levels with medication or vitamins will also lower the risk.
- *Fibrinogen*: another protein that, when elevated, can lead to an increased risk of clotting.
- *Infectious agents* (such as viruses and bacteria): chronic infection leads to chronic inflammation, which increases the risk of heart attack and stroke.
- *Lipoprotein (a) (LPa)*: a "bad" cholesterol particle that increases the risk of heart attack and stroke. LPa contributes to atherosclerotic

plaque formation and also increases the risk of blood clotting.

- *High sensitivity C-reactive protein (hs–CRP)*: a marker of inflammation that is linked to an increased risk of cardiovascular disease. Several studies have shown that hs-CRP is a better predictor of heart attack than total cholesterol or bad (LDL) cholesterol.
- *Particle size*: the size of the particles that carry cholesterol. This can be more important in predicting heart attack risk than the cholesterol level itself. Small bad (LDL) cholesterol particles are more dangerous than large bad cholesterol particles. Likewise, small good (HDL) cholesterol particles are less effective in removing bad (LDL) cholesterol particles from the blood vessel wall than large good (HDL) cholesterol particles.

Collectively, all of the risk factors mentioned above, along with other emerging risk factors, are termed "the atherogenic metabolic stew." These metabolic risk factors can be measured by most commercial labs. The task of the preventive cardiologist is to treat all of the known risk factors, thereby decreasing this deadly stew. This will result in a decrease in atherosclerotic plaque buildup as well as a decrease in the risk of heart attack, stroke, and peripheral vascular disease.

Important Medications for Cardiovascular Disease Prevention

Cardiovascular disease prevention begins with lifestyle modification. A proper diet and exercise program, along with stress management and smoking cessation, form the foundation of our heart disease prevention guidelines. There are people who nevertheless develop heart disease, even though they follow these guidelines. These individuals have a genetic basis for their heart disease, and require medications along with a healthy lifestyle.

Many types of medications are used in the treatment of cardiovascular disease. The most commonly used medications for cardiovascular disease prevention are listed below.

- *HMG-CoA reductase inhibitors (also known as statins)*: medications that reduce cholesterol levels by decreasing the production of cholesterol in the body. Clinical trials that have evaluated the impact of statins on heart disease prevention have demonstrated a significant lowering of heart attack risk and death from coronary heart disease.
- *Niacin, fibrates, resins, and cholesterol absorption inhibitors*: medications that can also lower cholesterol and triglyceride levels.
- *ACE inhibitors*: medications that lower blood pressure and help sta-

bilize the blood vessel wall. They have been shown to lower heart attack risk in patients with heart disease risk factors.

- *Beta blockers*: medications that decrease blood pressure and heart rate by blocking adrenaline. These drugs are especially useful in patients who have high blood pressure and cardiac arrhythmias (heart rhythm disorder). In addition, beta blockers have been shown to reduce the risk of sudden death in certain high-risk patients. Finally, beta blockers have also been shown to be useful in the treatment of congestive heart failure.

- *Aspirin*: a medication that decreases the risk of heart attack and stroke by blocking the effects of platelets, which are cells that contribute to thrombus (clot formation). Low-dose aspirin appears to be as effective as high-dose aspirin for cardiovascular protection. Unless there is a good reason not to, most physicians advise all patients with cardiovascular disease to take aspirin on a regular basis. In men and women without cardiovascular disease, low-dose aspirin has been shown to reduce the risk of heart attack in men over the age of fifty and reduce the risk of stroke in women over the age of sixty-five. As always, you should discuss the risks and benefits of aspirin therapy with your physician.

Many other medications are used in cardiovascular disease prevention. Calcium channel blockers and angiotensin receptor blockers, for instance, are blood pressure medications used to treat patients with cardiovascular disease. New medications are constantly being developed to battle heart disease. A more efficient good (HDL) cholesterol, developed through genetic engineering, could help to reverse heart disease by decreasing plaque buildup in our arteries.

It is very important to become knowledgeable about all the medications used to treat cardiovascular disease, and it is equally important to understand all of their potential side effects. There is no substitute for regular medical follow-up and discussion between you and your doctor about the medications that are best for your cardiovascular health.

Tips on Purchasing, Preparing, and Eating Foods in the Miami Mediterranean Diet

Olive Oil

People who live in the Mediterranean grow up with the taste of their local olive oil ingrained in their senses. When you consume a local oil, you can almost smell the soil and envision the tree that produced its fruit.

Buying olive oil can be both exciting and confusing because of the vast variety of oils available in supermarkets and specialty food markets. There are emerald green-colored oils and golden oils. There are virgin oils and pure oils. The oils come packaged in different shapes and sizes, from exquisite glass bottles to metal tins and even plastic containers. So how does one even start to make a selection?

Olive oils range from pale yellow to a deep, cloudy green. One can easily assume that the green oil is from green, barely ripe olives, but its color is often actually an indication that the oil has a wonderfully fresh, intensely fruity taste. The color yellow, however, does usually mean that the olives were picked late in the season, when black and ripe, often resulting in a sweeter, rounder flavor.

There are various grades of olive oil:

- *Extra-virgin olive oil*: obtained from the first pressing of the olive; has less than 1% acidity
- *Fine virgin olive oil*: obtained from the second pressing of the olives; usually made from slightly riper olives than extra-virgin olive oil; has a slightly higher level of acidity, about 1.5%
- *Refined olive oil*: created by using chemicals to extract the oil from the olives; a basically tasteless olive oil with an acidity level higher than 3.2%
- *Pure olive oil*: a blend of refined and virgin olive oils which is lighter in color and blander in taste than virgin olive oil; an all-purpose olive oil; the word "pure" simply refers to the fact no oils other than olive oil have been added

Virgin olive oil has more antioxidant properties than refined olive oil, and tends to raise good (HDL) cholesterol more effectively than refined olive oil. People with high cholesterol who replace the saturated fat in their diet with olive oil, particularly virgin olive oil, decrease their total cholesterol and bad (LDL) cholesterol.

Bulk oils are generally blends of olive oils from either a particular region or country, or sometimes even from different countries. They are blended together by manufacturing companies and sold in large-quantity tins, plastic bottles, even pails, that range in size from 1 gallon to as much as 55 gallons. This does not mean that they are inferior oils; however, these oils are not the special quality first, cold-pressed olive oils, which can be as expensive as very fine wines. All olive oils have the same amounts of monounsaturated and polyunsaturated fats (good fats); however, first cold-pressed olive oil will have more naturally occurring antioxidants than the regular-pressed olive oils. Blended bulk oils are sometimes a blend of first cold-pressed and regular-pressed oils. They still provide some of the health benefits of a pure first cold-pressed olive oil, but can be sold at a cheaper price.

When you buy olive oil, consider how you will use it. If you want to make a pasta sizzle, a young, peppery Tuscan oil might be your best bet, whereas a good, cured, full-bodied oil would be appropriate for a traditional Greek salad made of the best quality tomatoes and finest feta available. However, if you want a hint of olive oil with a background flavor, then a light fruity olive oil, perhaps one from Liguria or Provence that adds a layer of flavor but does not stand out, would be the way to go.

A few other tips:

- Olive oil far exceeds the health benefits of other oils, butters, margarines, or lard; it should be used to replace these items, not in conjunction with them.
- If an oil smells or tastes rancid, that usually indicates that it has been exposed to sunlight or another source of light, which reduces olive oil's delicate aromatic qualities and vitamin E content.
- When selecting an oil, look for the harvest date on the bottle. No olive oil improves with age; it should be no more than eighteen months old.
- An excellent olive oil can range from thirty to forty dollars a bottle, or as high as eighty dollars a bottle, much like an expensive bottle of wine of corresponding quality.
- Heating olive oil, especially at high temperatures as in deep frying, can decrease the levels of antioxidants in the oil.

Canola Oil

Canola oil is another heart-healthy oil. The word "canola" in "canola oil" comes from the words "Canada" and "oil"; it was developed in Canada during the late 1960s and early 1970s. It comes from a genetically engineered hybrid plant developed from different mustard seed plants and the turnip rapeseed.

Canola oil contains essential fatty acids which have been proven beneficial to health. Canola oil has zero trans fat, and high levels of heart-healthy monounsaturated fats and omega-3 fat.

Beans

Humble bean dishes are a staple in the Mediterranean, made with grains and an abundance of vegetables. On wintry days, throughout the countryside you can smell the delicious aroma of hearty bean soups that have been simmering for days. Beans are served hot or cold, as a first course or as a main dish, as part of a stew or perhaps a dip, to be scooped up with bread or vegetables—there are so many delicious ways in which they can be served.

But the best thing about beans is how healthy they are. They're high in complex carbohydrates, amino acids, fiber, iron, and folic acid. They contain little to no fat and no cholesterol, but an abundance of soluble fiber, which benefits our hearts by lowering cholesterol levels. They are also an excellent low-fat source of protein.

A good rule of thumb for purchasing beans is to buy only beans that are smooth and bright in color; beans that appear cracked, dull, and/or wrinkled are old, and the older the bean, the longer the cooking time needed. One cup of dry beans equals two to two and a half cups of cooked beans. Most dried beans must be soaked before they are cooked; the only exception is lentils.

There are two methods you can use for soaking beans: the power-soak method and the long-soak method. In the power-soak method, dried beans are boiled in water for about three minutes, then covered and set aside for two to four hours. After four hours the water is drained off and discarded, and the beans are rinsed under fresh running water. The beans are then returned to a heavy-bottomed pot, covered with fresh water, and cooked per package directions.

In the long-soak method, the beans are soaked for eight hours or more. After the required soaking time the water covering the beans is also discarded. As in the power-soak method, the beans are rinsed under fresh water then returned to a heavy-bottomed pot with fresh water and cooked per package directions.

With either method of soaking, you can test that a bean has been adequately soaked simply by cutting the bean in half to check its color. If the center is opaque, the beans need to be soaked longer. A bean is fully cooked when it can be mashed with a fork.

Below are a few major beans used in the Mediterranean region. Note that the following soaking instructions are for beans cooked in a pressure cooker; cooking beans in a pressure cooker requires less soaking time than conventional stovetop cooking.

Cannellini Bean: one of the most popular beans used in cuisines of central Italy. The cannellini bean is a small white kidney-shaped bean that is high in protein. These beans are great in soups and salads as well as by themselves with just a little olive oil drizzled over them. Soaking time is about 1½ hours (use a ratio of 1 cup of beans to 3 cups of water). One half (½) cup of cooked cannellini beans is roughly 100 calories.

Fava Bean (white or brown; also called the "broad bean"): a bean that goes back almost to the beginning of Mediterranean agriculture. Fava beans have tough outer skins (which are usually discarded after soaking) and a sweet, nutty-flavored inner taste. They are great in soups and salads, and are often used for dips and pâté. Soaking time is about 3 hours (use a ratio of 1 cup of beans to 4 cups of water). One half (½) cup of fava beans is roughly 93 calories.

Chickpea or Garbanzo Bean: another Old World bean with a long history in Mediterranean agriculture. Chickpeas are an excellent source of protein and iron. In North African regions they are used to make hummus. Soaking time is about 3 hours (use a ratio of 1 cup of beans to 4 cups of water). One half (½) cup of cooked chickpeas is roughly 130 calories.

Navy Bean: a member of the white bean family. These beans are great in soups and salads, and also stand alone well just in an oil-and-vinegar marinade. Soaking time is about 2 ½ hours (use a ratio of 1 cup of beans to 4 cups of water). One half (½) cup of cooked navy beans is roughly 130 calories.

Great Northern Bean: also a member of the white bean family, similar in flavor to the navy bean but larger in size. These beans do well in many dishes, as well as in an oil-and-vinegar marinade. Soaking time is about 2 hours (use a ratio of 1 cup of beans to 3 cups of water). One half (½) cup of cooked great northern is roughly 100 calories.

Lentil (brown, red, or green): a staple in many Mediterranean cuisines. Brown and green lentils do well in salads, whereas red ones are better suited for pâté and soups. Note: never substitute Indian lentils in a Mediterranean dish. Indian lentils are meant to disintegrate into a thick sauce upon cooking, and in Mediterranean cuisine, the lentils are meant to remain intact. No soaking is required. One half (½) cup of cooked red or brown lentils is roughly 120 calories. One half (½) cup of cooked green lentils is roughly 110 calories.

Some favorite spices used in France and Italy to flavor beans include rosemary, fennel, sage, caraway, tarragon, and marjoram. Lighter spices often include bay leaves, garlic, oregano, parsley, thyme, and dill. In the Middle Eastern countries stronger spices such as cumin, cinnamon, mint, and coriander prevail; on the lighter end, garlic, ginger, nutmeg, fresh pepper, marjoram, parsley, cilantro, saffron, paprika, and turmeric are often used.

A few hints for basic bean seasoning: When using chopped onions, garlic cloves, bay leaves, and cumin, cook them with the beans from the start. Wait until the beans are almost done before adding major seasonings. Adding spices too soon can cause them to break down and disappear before the meal is served.

Bean-related flatulence can be a major problem for some people. Many beans contain a sugar molecule called oligosaccharides. When bacteria breaks down this sugar molecule in the large intestine, it causes flatulence as a by-product. To reduce the occurrence of flatulence, never use the same water that the beans have been soaking in to also cook the beans; always discard soaking water, rinse beans, and cook in fresh water. By soaking the beans for several hours and then discarding the water, you soak off and get rid of some of the offending sugars, reducing the problem of flatulence and possibly eliminating it completely.

Grains

Grains, which make up the foundation of the Mediterranean diet, appear at almost every meal in one form or another. They provide the bulk of the Mediterranean diet's protein and many of its calories, and in the form of complex carbohydrates are the perfect energy source.

Grains can be divided into two groups: whole grains (the grains commonly used in a traditional Mediterranean diet) and refined grains. Whole grains include the entire grain kernel, consisting of the bran, the germ, and the endosperm. Refined grains are whole grains that have been milled, a process that destroys the bran and germ of the kernel, removing dietary fiber, iron, and B-vitamins. Refining gives grains a smoother texture and makes them last longer on the shelf, which is why it has become a common practice in the United States. Many refined grains have been "enriched," meaning that iron and some vitamins have been put back into the product, but the fiber cannot be replaced.

The following are some of the most commonly used grains.

Wheat

Wheat is one of the cornerstones of the Mediterranean diet, in the form of bread, pasta, couscous, and bulgur. There are many types of wheat ranging from very soft wheat (*Triticum aestivum*) to very hard wheat (*Triticum durum*). The terms "soft" and "hard" do not refer to the texture of the wheat but to the protein content of the wheat: hard wheat is generally higher both in protein and in the gluten needed for bread making (gluten is responsible for the stretchiness of dough). Soft wheat is most often used for commercial pizza dough and pastries.

Durum hard grain is the hardest wheat grown. Although it is a soft creamy yellow in color, its texture is coarser than regular wheat flour. When durum wheat is milled—when the outer portions of the wheat are stripped away, leaving only its heart—the result is called semolina flour. Golden in color, semolina flour has an even higher proportion of protein and gluten content than whole durum, and is used almost exclusively for pasta production; in Morocco, it is also used to make couscous and homemade breads.

Bread

Semolina flour is often used to make bread, sometimes alone but usually combined with unbleached or all-purpose flour. The best all-purpose flour is a blend of hard and soft wheat that is unbleached and unbromated. ("Unbleached" means that the flour has not been treated with chemicals such as chlorine or peroxide to make it whiter; "unbromated" means the flour has not been enriched using chemicals like potassium bromate.) Most health food stores carry at least one unbleached and unbromated type of all-purpose flour.

Whole wheat flour, another great flour for bread making, is flour that contains the whole wheat kernel, or berry. The amount of husk and wheat germ retained by the flour varies depending upon how it is milled; a flour's performance, flavor, and nutrition are greatly affected by the type of mill that grinds the grain. Whole wheat flour, for instance, is stone-ground.

Stone-ground mills produce the best flour, because they do not overheat it as in other milling methods, instead flaking layers off the grain. This results in more of the nutrients being retained in the flour.

Pasta

Pasta comes in many shapes, flavors, and textures, but shares the same basic ingredients: flour and water. The best industrial pasta is made from semolina flour, because it absorbs much less water than other flours. That's why pastas imported from Italy are usually of such high quality—the pastas usually list durum wheat flour or semolina among their ingredients.

One pound of pasta generally feeds six people as an appetizer or four people as a main course. Two ounces of uncooked pasta generally equals one cup of cooked pasta. When pairing sauces with pastas, generally pureed, creamy, or clinging sauces are best served with thin strands of pasta like spaghetti, fettuccine, cappellini, or linguine, because they will allow the sauce to flow evenly over the noodle. Thinner, runnier sauces are better held by pastas that have twisted or curled shapes because they trap the liquid, making sure the sauce coats the pasta rather than the plate, whereas chunky sauces go best with chunky pastas, particularly ones that contain an opening, like elbow macaroni or shell pastas. Tiny pastas like orzo are great with just a little olive oil and herbs; rich sauces tend to overwhelm them.

Tips for cooking pasta:

- Use three quarts of rapidly boiling water for ½ pound of pasta and four quarts for one pound of pasta.
- Make sure your pot is large and roomy.
- Salt the water before adding pasta, not after (generally one teaspoon of salt per ½ pound of pasta).
- Do not stir noodles that stick to the bottom of the pot; instead, gently lift them with a fork.
- Check pasta at two to four minutes for thin pasta and eight to ten minutes for denser pasta.
- Drain pasta once it's finished cooking but do not rinse; this keeps the pasta moist and helps the sauce stick.
- Add sauce immediately after draining and serve. If not serving im-

mediately, toss pasta with one to two tablespoons of olive oil; this will prevent pasta from sticking.

- If you're making a pasta salad, put dressing on hot noodles immediately to let it sink in; the starchiness of the hot pasta helps the sauce cling to the noodles.
- If pasta is going to be cooked further, such as in a baked dish, undercook it slightly when boiling. This is called cooking it *al dente*.

Various sizes and shapes of pastas:

Shaped pasta: pastas in shapes such as shells, bow ties, spirals, wheels, and curly shapes. The smaller of these varieties do best with a simple, plain sauce; however, the larger ones can usually handle a thicker, chunkier sauce because they are sturdier. Some examples:

- Cavatelli shells (small, narrow shells)
- Conchigliette (medium-sized shells)
- Fusilli (short, twisted, curly pastas)
- Gnocchi shells (small shells made from potato dough)
- Ruotine (small wheels)
- Fusilli (spirals)
- Farfalle (bow ties)

Tubular pastas: any pastas in the shape of a tube, from short and wide to long and narrow. The outside can be smooth or textured, and be cut off straight or at an angle. These pastas are hearty and can handle very chunky, thick sauces, which cling well to both the insides and outside of the pasta. The larger varieties of these tubular pastas are great for stuffing with meat and/or cheese. Some examples:

- Penne (two-inch long smooth tubes)
- Rigatoni (thick tubes that can be two inches long or longer, often with outside grooves)
- Ziti (straight or slightly curved tubes, either smooth or grooved on the outside)
- Cannelloni (very large tubes; great for stuffing)

- Manicotti (very large tubes, slightly smaller than Cannelloni, that often come flat for rolling; also great for stuffing)

Strand pastas: long rods of pasta which come in a variety of thickness, from very long and thin to very short and thick. The thicker kinds do well with heavy sauces, whereas the very thin kinds require light, plain sauces. Some examples:

- Spaghetti (long rods of various medium thicknesses)
- Capellini, or angel hair (long, very thin rods)
- Vermicelli (long round rods somewhere in thickness between a thinner spaghetti and capellini)
- Linguine (long, flat, thin pasta)
- Tagliateline (long, flat, thin pasta slightly wider than linguine)
- Fettuccine (long, flat, thin pasta wider than both linguine and tagliateline)

Ribbon pastas: long flat pieces of pasta which come in a variety of lengths and widths; can be curled or straight on the sides. These pastas are generally used with a thick sauce. Some examples:

- Lasagna (long rectangular pieces roughly 2–3 inches wide and curly on both side edges)
- Tagliatelle (long rectangular pieces roughly 1 inch wide and curly on both side edges)
- Papparelle (long rectangular pieces about 1–1½ inches wide and curly on both side edges)

Soup pastas: small to tiny pastas, most frequently used in soups, that come in a variety of shapes. The larger of the small size can be used with thicker soups while the tiny ones are better in a thinner broth. Shapes include flat pieces, balls, tubes, rings, stars, grain shapes, thin strands, and even letters or numbers. Some examples:

- Orzo (small rice-shaped pasta)
- Ditalini (tiny tubes less than ¼-inch long)
- Tubettini (very tiny tubes, smaller than ditalini)

- Alfabeto (alphabet-shaped pasta)
- Anchellini (thin, short, flat pieces of pasta)

Because pastas come in many shapes and flavors, their caloric value per cup varies greatly.

The key to keeping pasta a healthy low-fat food is to use whole grain pasta and to not top with a rich, fatty sauce.

Couscous

What pasta is to the Italians and rice is to the Chinese, couscous is to the inhabitants of Morocco, Algeria, and Tunisia; it's used to make appetizers, soups, salads, main course dishes, and even desserts. When entering a kitchen during mealtime it's quite common to see a steaming platter of couscous topped with vegetables, meat, or fish. Couscous is often eaten with only vegetables and perhaps goat cheese and/or nuts. When meat is used, it is usually lamb, chicken, or pork.

Couscous is made from durum wheat. The wheat is milled into semolina, rolled into thin strands, crumbled into tiny pieces, steamed, and dried. (Unlike pasta, it is not kneaded during the semolina-water mixture stage.) The word "couscous" refers both to this dry semolina product and the popular prepared dish in which it is the principal ingredient.

The coarsest, largest size of couscous is used primarily for soups. Medium-sized couscous, which is mostly what we see here in the United States, is all-purpose. Tiny or ant-sized couscous is reserved for special dishes and desserts.

When convenience is needed, pre-steamed couscous is used. Pre-steamed couscous greatly reduces the final cooking time for a dish, since it needs only fifteen minutes in boiling liquid before it is ready to serve.

Bulgur

Bulgur is commonly used in salad preparations, but most often used to make Tabbouleh. It is made by cracking parboiled whole wheat kernels (kernels boiled until they are partially cooked) and drying them. Bulgur wheat does not need to be cooked, but should be soaked in warm water for twenty to thirty minutes (to soften it) before using. However, when making pilaf (another popular use for bulgur), you don't need to soak the bulgur before using it—you are cooking all the ingredients together at the same time, and the bulgur will soften during that process.

Rice

Worldwide, rice is the most consumed food, eaten by millions every day. In the Mediterranean diet, rice is as popular as wheat flour, and in some regions it's even preferred. In the regions of the western Mediterranean, it takes the form of dishes like risotto and paella. In Greece, Turkey, and the Levant, it shows up as long-grain rice, originally from India and Persia, and is used to make pilaf (long-grain rice makes a better paella because it cooks up dry and fluffy, whereas short-grain rice becomes tender and sticky when cooked). Brown rice, unquestionably a healthier product, is not often used in the Mediterranean except by people eating a macrobiotic diet.

To cook most rice, use a ratio of 1 cup of rice to 1½ or 2 cups of water. Put the rice in a heavy pot with water and salt and cover with a tight-fitting lid; bring to a boil, then reduce heat to medium-low and let simmer for 1 hour, or until water is completely absorbed. Finally, when the time is up, keep the pot covered tightly for another 10 minutes before serving.

Polenta

Polenta is a favorite dish in northern Italy, where it is cooked in water and then eaten with a drizzle of olive oil and a sprinkle of Parmesan cheese, or with tomato sauce. It is a traditional dish and often replaces rice, pasta, or potatoes.

Polenta is made of gluten-free, coarsely ground cornmeal that is either white or yellow in color, rather like semolina in appearance. The best polenta is stone-ground cornmeal, where the whole grain, including the germ, is retained.

Fish

In the past decade one of the single most important health recommenda tions has been to increase our dietary intake of omega-3 fatty acids. Numerous scientific studies tout their health: they have been shown to reduce blood pressure and systemic and vascular inflammation, and decrease triglyceride levels and heart rhythm disturbances. Consequently, omega-3 fatty acids may be helpful in treating or improving a wide variety of diseases, such as rheumatoid arthritis, inflammatory bowel diseases, periodontal diseases, depression, acne, asthma, and other disorders.

Cold water fish is rich in EPA and DHA, two omega-3 fatty acids that have been proven beneficial to heart health. But that's not all fish has to offer. Fish is an excellent source of protein, and lower in calories than other meat sources. Fish is also lower in fat, particularly cholesterol and saturated fat.

The American Heart Association states that "eating a variety of fish is beneficial to fetal development in pregnant women." However, pregnant women (and children) should avoid certain species of fish (swordfish, shark, tilefish, and king mackerel) as these large predatory fish may contain higher levels of environmental contaminants like mercury. Because of the mercury content of some fish, it is recommended that the skin of the fish be removed before cooking—higher levels of mercury may be concentrated in the skin.

The chart below provides a general overview of the omega-3 content of some popular varieties of finfish (fish with a bony skeleton) and shellfish, based on a 3-ounce raw edible portion for finfish and a 3 ½-ounce raw edible portion for shellfish.

Fish Omega-3/mg

Catfish, channel or farmed 373	Mackerel, Atlantic 2299
Cod, Atlantic............................184	Mackerel, Pacific 1442
Cod, Pacific....... 215	Ocean Perch 289
Dolphin; Mahi-mahi...............108	Perch 253
Flounder; Sole 199	Pollack, Atlanta 421
Grouper, mixed species............248	Pompano, Florida....................568
Haddock 185	Sablefish 1395
Hake 225	Salmon, Atlantic....................1435
Halibut, Atlantic and Pacific ...495	Salmon, King Chinook 1355
Herring, Atlantic....................1571	Salmon, Sockeye....................1200
Herring, Pacific 1658	Sea bass, mixed species 590

Sea trout, mixed species...........373
Shark, mixed species................845
Snapper, mixed species 311
Swordfish 639
Trout, Rainbow.......................568

Tuna, Blue Fin.......................1173
Tuna, Skipjack.........................256
Tuna, Yellow Fin......................218
Turbot, Greenland...................920
Whitefish, mixed species 1258

Shellfish Omega-3/mg

Clams, mixed species...............142
Crab, Alaska King 400
Crab, Blue...............................320
Crab, Dungeness......................400
Crab, Queen 375
Crawfish, mixed species...........175
Lobster...................................373

Mussels...................................440
Octopus 150
Oysters...................................678
Scallops, mixed species 198
Shrimp, mixed species 480
Squid, mixed species...............488

Nuts

Nut consumption has been shown to be beneficial for cardiovascular health and to reduce the risk of heart attack. Several landmark studies have revealed the importance of regular nut consumption:

- The Adventist Health Study of 31,000 men and women in 1992 at Loma Linda University in California showed that those who consumed nuts more than five times a week had up to 60% fewer heart attacks than those who ate nuts less than once monthly.
- Harvard Men's Health Watch showed that healthy men and men who have suffered a heart attack can actually decrease their cardiovascular risk by eating nuts on a regular basis.
- Iowa Women's Healthy Study in 1996, involving more than 34,000 postmenopausal women, found that those who ate nuts more than four times a week were 40% less likely to die of heart disease.
- Physician's Health Study in 2002 found that men who consumed nuts two or more times per week had reduced risk of sudden cardiac death.

Nuts are a great source of protein and are rich in fiber. In addition, they contain phytonutrients and antioxidants such as vitamin E and selenium.

They are high in plant sterol, but mostly contain healthy monounsaturated and polyunsaturated fats like omega-3 that have been shown to lower bad (LDL) cholesterol. As little as two ounces of nuts a week may help lower heart disease risk.

If you are afraid the caloric content of nuts will make you gain weight (an ounce of nuts can contain more than 200 calories, after all), instead of simply adding nuts to your diet, eat them as a replacement for foods that are high in saturated fats and limit your intake to one or two ounces a day. For instance, don't add chocolate chips or icing to cookies; instead, sprinkle on some nuts. Or instead of making a meat or cheese sandwich, try a nut-butter sandwich. In most markets today you can find several varieties of nut butters, from almond nut butter to cashew and even macadamia nut butter.

Peanut butter, of course, is another healthy choice; however, peanuts are not actually nuts, they're legumes. They are, however, as healthy a snack as nuts since they also contain fiber, micronutrients, and antioxidants that are essential for good health. Several studies involving peanuts, such as the ground-breaking Harvard School of Public Health Study, report that eating an ounce of nuts or one tablespoon of peanut butter five times or more a week reduced the risk of developing type II diabetes by 21 to 27%.

Purdue University conducted a study that found that peanuts and peanut butter produced greater feelings of satiety and fullness than other high-carbohydrate snacks. Peanuts kept the participants satisfied for as much as 2–2 ½ hours longer than other snacks. Furthermore, the participants self-adjusted their caloric intake after eating peanuts: they did not add extra calories to their daily intake. The Purdue University Study showed that nut- and peanut-eaters tend to have lower body mass index (BMI) than non-nut-eaters. It also showed that when people ate peanuts, they naturally decreased what they ate at other times of the day, resulting in improved weight control.

APPENDIX D

Eating Out on the Miami Mediterranean Diet (The Restaurant Survival Guide)

It's easy to follow the Miami Mediterranean diet at home, but what do you do when you're faced with a restaurant menu? Relax. You can take the Miami Mediterranean diet on the road and still have a great time. Just use these easy-to-follow guidelines:

- Don't go to a restaurant when you're starving. Drink a glass of water and enjoy a handful of almonds before you go. That way, you won't be tempted to devour the breadbasket while you're waiting for your meal.
- Speaking of that breadbasket, avoid it. Instead, ask to exchange it for whole grain bread and a small dish of olive oil (to be used sparingly on bread instead of margarine or butter). But remember, if you're watching your calories, a tablespoon of olive oil has 120 calories; be sure to use it in moderation.
- Choose fish or skinless poultry over red meat.
- Avoid foods that are fried; opt for grilled, baked, or broiled instead.
- Steer clear of processed or frozen food. Fresh food is healthier, and tastes much better.
- Be certain that food isn't cooked with trans fats (hydrogenated oils).

Ask to be sure!

- When ordering pasta, ask for whole grain.
- Order a salad with fresh vegetables and balsamic or olive oil dressing.
- Select brown rice instead of white rice.
- Avoid fruit drinks and sodas.
- Eat half your portion and take the rest home—in fact, ask for half of it to be wrapped up ahead of time, before it is even brought to the table!
- Order fresh fruit for dessert.
- Consider hot green tea after your meal.

Glossary

Al dente: Italian for pasta cooked until it is slightly resistant to the bite.

All-purpose flour: a blend of soft and hard wheat; the best type is unbleached.

Antioxidants: compounds that may have the potential to prevent numerous diseases by interfering with the cellular destruction caused by free radicals.

Basil: a very aromatic herb with a sweet, mildly pungent flavor that is widely used in Italy.

Bay leaf: another aromatic herb, with a slightly bitter taste; the greener the leaf, the more flavor it has. When fresh, the leaf is dark green on one side and lighter on the other. Properly dried bay leaf should be olive green in color.

Bruschetta: crusty slices of bread drenched with extra-virgin olive oil, rubbed with generous amounts of garlic, and grilled or toasted on both sides.

Bulgur: whole wheat kernels that are steamed, dried, and crushed. Bulgur has a tender, chewy consistency, and comes in three grades: coarse, medium, and fine. The coarser size is best for pilaf, while the medium size is good for Tabbouleh.

Calorie: a unit of heat energy that expresses the energy exchanges of the body and the potential energy values of food.

Canola/olive oil spread: trans fat–free, plant-based buttery spreads that can be used to replace butter and other buttery products, which often contain saturated fat and even trans fats. Examples of plant-based spreads include Smart Balance and Promise.

Carbohydrates: the source of energy gained from food; they can be either complex or simple.

Cayenne: the dried, powdered fruit of the red hot pepper. It is much like paprika in appearance and is used in small amounts to give a fiery kick to many dishes.

Cholesterol: a type of fat derived from animal sources. Cholesterol is transported through the body by carriers called lipoproteins. Excessive amounts of cholesterol circulating in the blood can build up on artery walls and eventually lead to heart attack and stroke.

Cilantro: a very pungent herb; part of the parsley family, and often used instead of parsley in dishes where a stronger accent is desired.

Complex carbohydrates: energy-yielding nutrients which provide the most efficient fuel source for the body. Complex carbohydrates metabolize more slowly than simple carbohydrates, providing the body with energy over a longer period of time. Examples of complex carbohydrates are legumes, vegetables, and whole grains.

Cornmeal: a white or yellow grain (though yellow is more typical) which has a grainy texture and a sweet taste. In Italy cornmeal is called polenta.

Couscous: a type of pasta made from semolina and water. What rice is in China, couscous is in Morocco, Algeria, and Tunisia. Couscous is now available in an instant form, which just needs to be covered with boiling water.

Crostini: thin slices of crusty bread baked in an oven at 350 degrees until golden in color, rubbed with garlic, and drenched in extra-virgin olive oil.

Cumin: a dried, slightly bitter fruit that is part of the parsley family. It has a strong scent and flavor.

Dietary fiber: the parts of fruits and vegetables and whole grains that are not digested or absorbed by the body. There are two types of dietary fiber: soluble and insoluble. Soluble fiber forms a jell-like mass around food parts and helps to prevent the absorption of cholesterol by promoting its excretion. Insoluble fibers add bulk to stools and help you feel satiated.

Durum flour: flour ground from durum wheat. Durum flour is very fine flour that is very high in gluten.

Fat: one of three main classes of nutrients that provide energy to the body. Fats are either saturated or unsaturated.

Feta cheese: cheese made from pasteurized sheep's or goat's milk.

Focaccia: an Italian oven-baked round or rectangular bread filled with herbs, onions, spices, and often an array of vegetables.

Free radicals: unstable products of metabolism that have a destructive effect on cells' DNA. The damaged DNA not only suppresses the immune system but has also been implicated in the development of many diseases, such as heart disease, cancer, and other chronic illnesses.

Garlic: a member of the onion family with a distinctively rich, hot flavor (though the flavor can be mild or strong, depending on how it is sliced or chopped and how long it is cooked). Garlic has been shown to have beneficial effects on blood pressure, cholesterol, and other risk factors.

Gluten: a protein substance (especially of wheat flour) that gives cohesiveness to dough.

Harissa, hareesa, or hreesa: a fiery hot paste made by pounding together red chili peppers, spices, and olive oil. It is used to season couscous and many North African dishes.

Italian frittatas: savory omelets cooked into a thick cake brimming with potatoes and onions or other vegetables. It is most delicious when served warm from the oven.

Kesra: a dense round loaf of bread predominately seen in the Northwestern African regions, largely Morocco, Algeria, and Tunisia. Kesra is flavored with whole aniseeds or sesame seeds and is great for dipping in soups or eating with stews.

Khubz: Arab pita bread used to scoop up sauces, dips, yogurts, and liquids, or cut in half and filled with shish kabobs, falafel, or salads. Arabs eat bread with every meal, and consider bread to be a divine gift from God.

Lavosh: a very crispy flat Egyptian bread.

Lipoproteins: combinations of fat and protein that transport lipids (fats) in the blood.

Low-calorie baking sweeteners: refined sugar substitutes that do well in recipes when the recipe calls for heat, such as in baking and cooking. These products usually have ½ or less than ½ the calories of refined sugar.

Mediterranean crusty country bread: a favorite, hearty, slightly sour crusty bread consumed throughout France, Italy, Spain, and Portugal.

Mint: an herb with a strong sweet aroma that is available fresh or dried. Also great as a garnish.

Monounsaturated fat: a naturally occurring heart-healthy fat found in plant foods. Research has found that monounsaturated fats actually play an important role in helping prevent heart disease and cancer. It is believed that it generally helps to maintain or raise good (HDL) cholesterol while decreasing bad (LDL) cholesterol. A few examples of foods high in monounsaturated fats are nuts, olives, and avocados.

Mozzarella: a soft spongy white cheese with a slightly sour flavor.

Non-caloric sweeteners: replacements for refined sugar that have no caloric value such as Splenda, Equal, Stevia, and Sweet'N Low.

Obesity: a condition in which a person exceeds the healthy weight for his or her height and body composition by 20% or more. The BMI, or body mass index, is used to define obesity. The BMI categories:

< 18.5	*underweight*
18.5–24.9	*normal weight*
25–29.9	*overweight*
> 30	*obese*

Oregano: a very popular Italian herb closely related to marjoram.

Paella: a variable Spanish rice dish often containing chicken, mussels, whitefish, peas, and rice, flavored with saffron, salt, pepper, and pimiento.

Parmesan cheese: a hard cheese made from semi-skim unpasteurized cow's milk.

Parsley: one of the most commonly used herbs. It adds both flavor and color to many dishes.

Pecorino: a sheep's milk cheese that has recently become more available in finer cheese shops here in the United States.

Pesto: a paste made from basil, olive oil, and pine nuts. The word comes from the Italian verb *pestare*, which means "to pound." It was often hand-made using a mortar and pestle to grind the herbs, lending a wonderful coarseness in texture. It was said that this assertive green sauce was a traditional favorite of Genoese sailors. In Italy, cooks are discreet with their pesto use; a little of this rich, highly flavored sauce goes a long way. Today, pre-made pesto sauces are available in most markets. The fresh pesto in tubs usually has more flavor then the jar varieties; however, nothing is as good as homemade.

Pistou: a pounded pesto-like sauce made of nuts, olive oil, garlic, and basil. It is unique to the Mediterranean region in France, and adds both body and herbaceous flavor to soups and stews.

Pita bread: a flat, round, hollow bread common to the cuisines of Africa and the Middle East.

Polenta: coarse-textured cornmeal. Pre-cooked instant polenta is now available in most markets, but does not taste as good as homemade polenta.

Polyunsaturated fat: highly unsaturated fats obtained from plants like corn, sunflower, and safflower oils that help reduce bad (LDL) cholesterol levels. They are also present in food such as oily fish, walnuts, and certain types of seeds.

Ratatouille: a vegetable casserole of tomatoes, eggplant, green peppers, zucchini, onions, and seasonings.

Risotto: an Italian rice dish made with butter, chopped onion, stock or wine, and Parmesan cheese. Meats or seafood and vegetables may also be added.

Saffron: a rather expensive dried yellow crocus native to the Mediterranean with a strong yellow color and a delicate flavor that is used in many Mediterranean dishes.

Saturated fat: a type of fat found in animal foods such as red meat and poultry, and dairy products, such as butter and whole milk. Other foods high in saturated fats include tropical cooking oils such as palm and coconut oils. High intakes of saturated fats have been linked to cardiovascular disease and cancer.

Semolina: roughly ground durum wheat used to make pasta and bread. It is technically not a grain but a nutritive tissue of durum wheat, the hardest of all wheat, and it is traditionally used to make pasta.

Simple carbohydrates: sugars which are quickly absorbed into the bloodstream, providing an immediate source of energy. Food sources like candy and soda are good examples of simple carbohydrates.

Sodium-free salt substitute: salt substitutes that contain either no sodium or reduced sodium content. Examples include No Salt and Salt Sense.

Soft and hard (wheat): this refers not just to the texture of the wheat but also to the protein content. Most hard wheat is higher in protein as well as in the gluten necessary for bread making.

Tahini: a paste made from crushed sesame seeds.

Tapas: Spanish appetizers, often called the "little dishes of Spain."

Trans fat: a type of fat found in stick margarine, vegetable shortening, and any food product that lists hydrogenated oils as one of its ingredients. The consumption of food products containing trans fats has been linked with the development of heart disease, diabetes, obesity, and cancer.

Turmeric: a relatively inexpensive rich yellow spice with flavoring similar to saffron that is used as a replacement for saffron in many dishes. It is a member of the ginger family.

Whole wheat flour: dark whole grain flour that has not had the bran and germ milled out of it. Some whole wheats are coarser than others. The best stone-ground whole wheat has a nutty wholesome flavor.

Whole wheat pastry flour: flour made from softer wheat that is more finely milled than whole wheat flour. In Italy it is used to make pizza and other pastries.

Recipe Index

Salads

Soups

Pizza, Pizza Sauces, and Pizza Crusts

Pizza

Side Dishes

Wraps and Sandwiches

Breads

Homemade Breads

Bread-Machine Breads

Desserts

Spices, Sauces, Marinades, and Dressings

Index

About the Author

MICHAEL OZNER, MD, FACC, FAHA, is one of America's leading advocates for heart disease prevention. Dr. Ozner is a board-certified cardiologist, a Fellow of the American College of Cardiology and of the American Heart Association, medical director of Wellness & Prevention at Baptist Health South Florida, and a well-known regional and national speaker in the field of preventive cardiology. He is the medical director of the Cardiovascular Prevention Institute of South Florida and symposium director for "Cardiovascular Disease Prevention," an annual international meeting highlighting advances in preventive cardiology. He was the recipient of the 2008 American Heart Association Humanitarian Award. Dr. Ozner is also the author of the BenBella Books title *The Great American Heart Hoax*.

To contact Dr. Michael Ozner: www.drozner.com